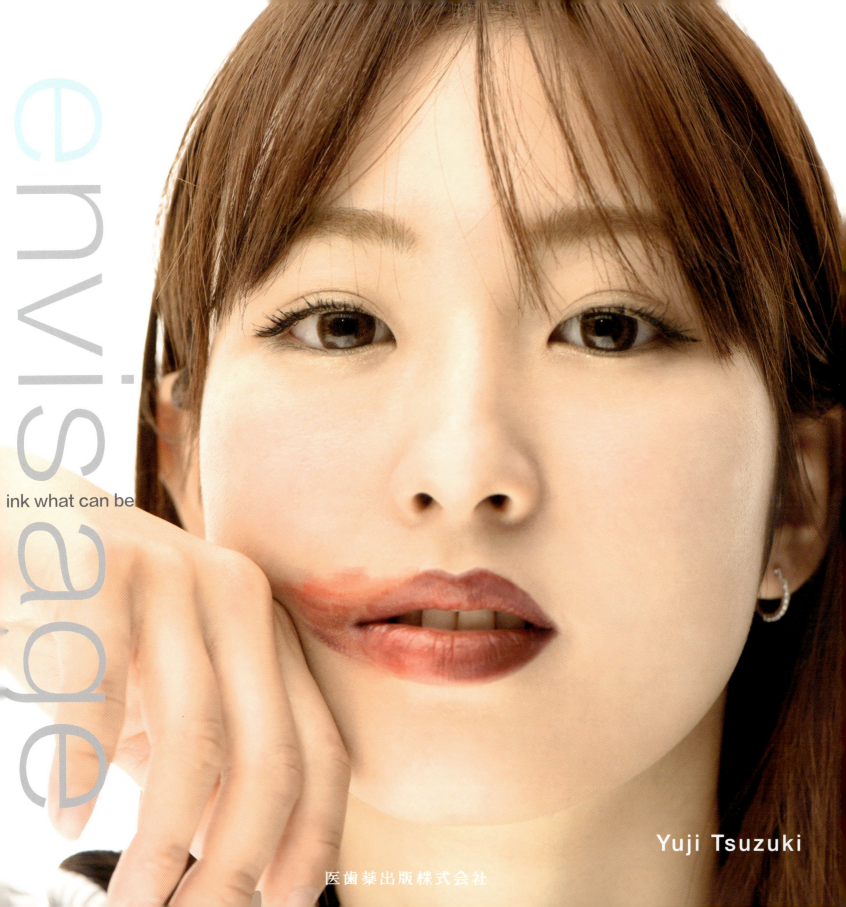

This book was originally published in Japanese
under the title of :

Envisage think what can be
Author :

YUJI, Tsuzuki

© 2019   1st ed.

ISHIYAKU PUBLISHERS, INC.
    7-10 Honkomagome 1 chome, Bunkyo-ku,
    Tokyo 113-8612, Japan

Prologue

歯科臨床に身を置き，早くも18年が経過した．

セラミックワークとの出会いは歯科技工士養成校を卒業後間もなく訪れ，その神秘的な再現技法に魅了された．そして，審美修復治療に携わる喜びや楽しさは，必然的に醒めることのない情熱へと変わっていった．

しかしながらその道のりは決して平坦なものではなく，どこか物足りなさを感じる日々も続いていた．そこには，何かしらの審美的要素を満たすエッセンスが欠如していたのだ．それは時に形態や色調の再現力であったり，歯列のバランス構成であったりした．また，技術的な問題とは別に，そもそもの修復条件さえ整っていないことに気付けないこともあった．

審美修復治療がもたらす結果は，患者のみならず術者にとっても大きな喜びを反映してくれるが，その反面，見た目の評価というものは残酷なまでに正直であった．

本書は，ここ10年を費やして撮り溜めた症例を一冊にまとめたものであるが，それぞれの治療背景や製作過程等を十分に想い浮かべながらご高覧いただければ幸いである．

口腔内印象が到着してから，模型上で想像を巡らせ製作した補綴装置が，わずかな緊張感を帯びながら口腔内へと装着される瞬間を，ぜひとも想い描いていただきたい．

そして，修復治療が無事完成にたどりつくためには，チェアサイドとの緊密な連携と相互の信頼関係が何よりも欠かせないということを感じ取っていただきたい．

そのうえで，審美修復治療の持つ可能性や趣を改めて感じ，歯科技工士として何ができるのか，また何をするべきなのか，読者諸氏にとってその道筋を心に明確に描くためのきっかけの一部となることを静かに願いたい．

そんな願いを込めた本書のタイトル『Envisage』であるが，セドナの広い夜空の下で林　直樹先生よりアドバイスをいただいたことを今でも鮮明に思い出す．常に，新たなチャレンジと指標を示して下さる林先生には，この場を借りて尊敬の念を伝えさせていただきます．

最後に，筆者をパートナーとして受け入れ，日常臨床からも多大な理解とご協力をいただいている歯科医師の先生方，そしてこれまでのRay Dental Laborを支えてくれたスタッフや関係者の皆様，また常に全力でサポートして下さるIvoclar Vivadent株式会社に心より感謝したい．

Ray Dental Labor
都築　優治

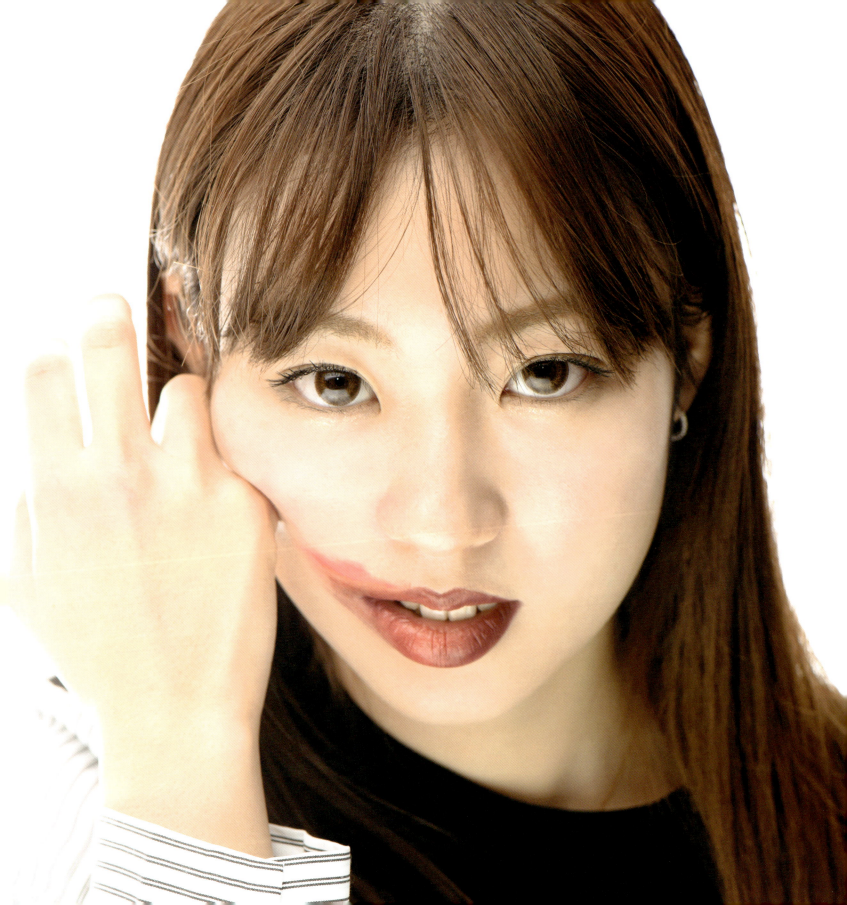

創造の世界へ・・・

envisage

think what can be

Contents

Prologue - 003

Case Gravures - 008

Part 1 : Mimicking Nature

Maxillary Single Central Incisor - 010

Part 2 : Individuality

Maxillary Central Incisors - 054

Part 3 : Harmony

between Esthetic and Function - 086

Part 4 : Creations

for a best smile : 106

Ceramic Works : 148

Behind the scenes - 176

Epilogue -186

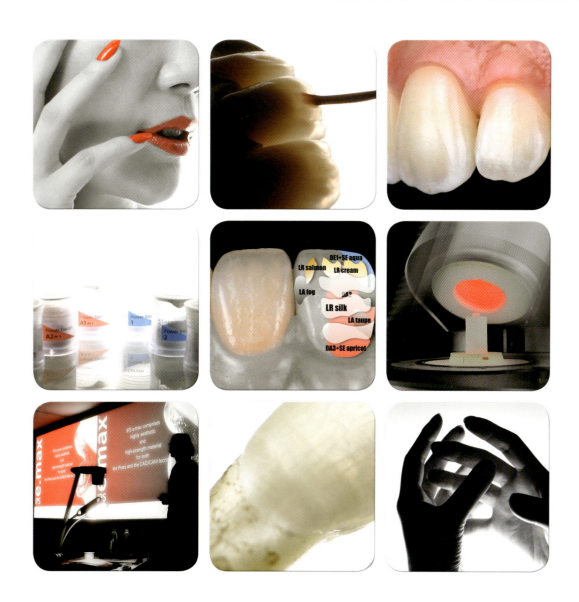

Designed by Yasunori SATO (a-pex design)

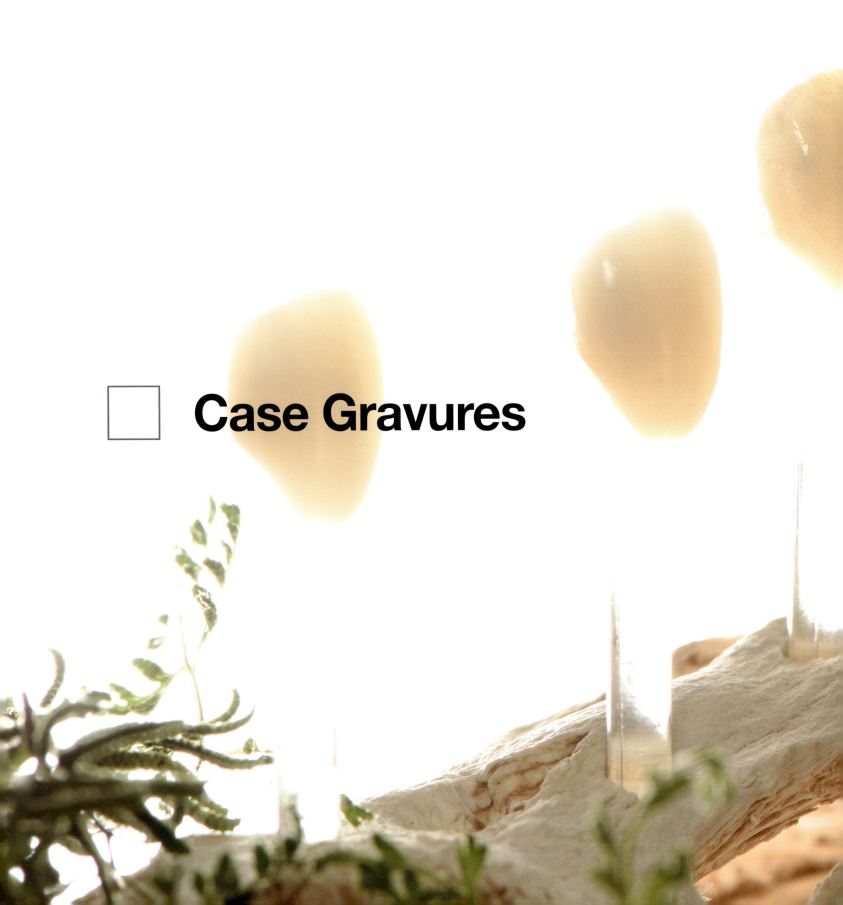

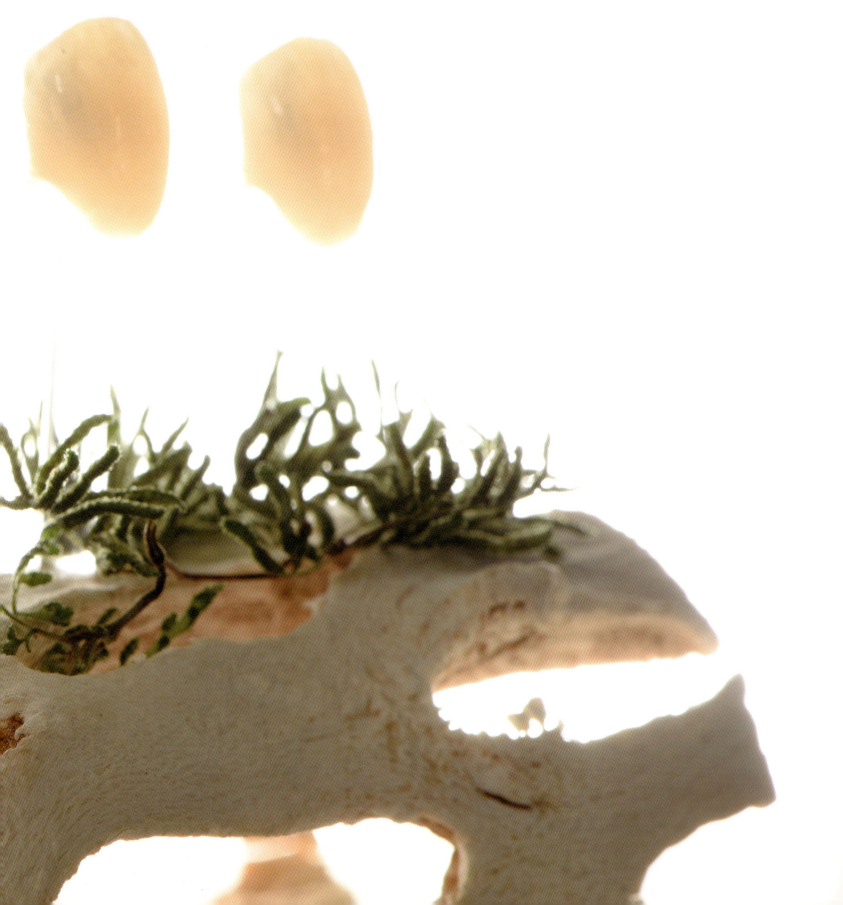

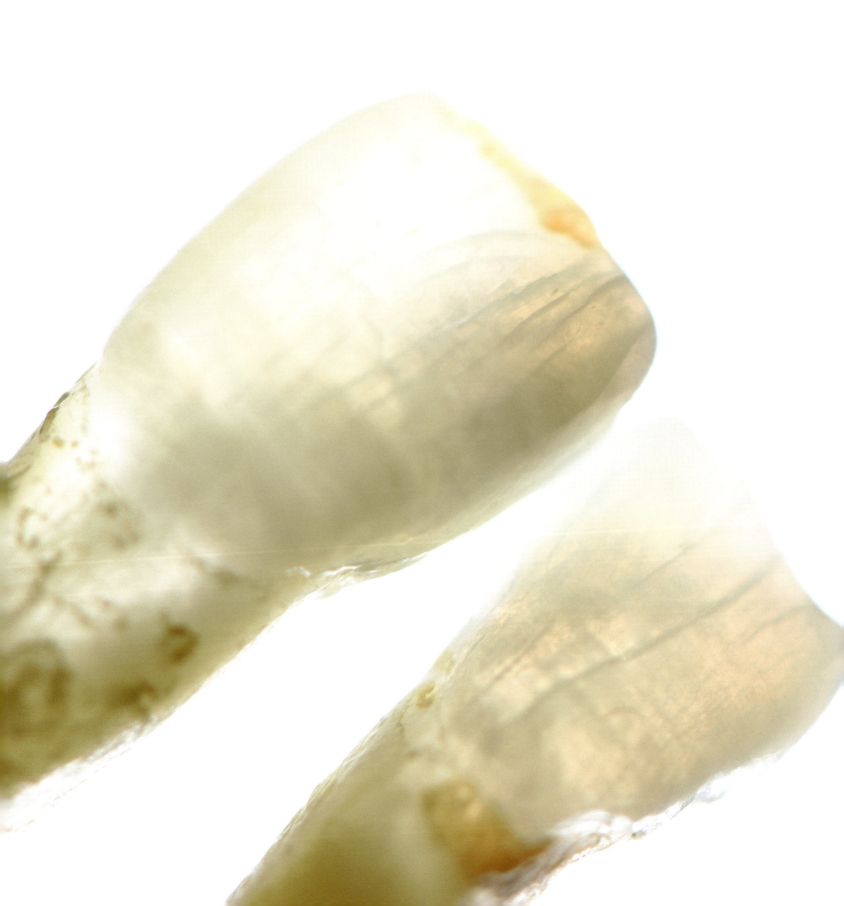

Part 1 : Mimicking Nature

Maxillary Single Central Incisor

「自然美の再現」

自然美の再現，それは飽くなき探求心から生まれる究極の成果である．
その中でも，上顎中切歯における模倣作業は，形態・色調・質感などすべて
の特徴を詳細に捉え，左右対称性に重きを置きながら微細な表現を積み重ね
ていかなければならない．そこには，高い再現力と色調の分析能力が欠かせ
ないが，自然に学び，その構造や成り立ちを理解することが成功への近道と
なる．
Digital Dentistry の発展に伴い，これまで集積されたテクノロジーや歯科解
剖学はいとも簡単に再現可能なものとなっている．
しかしながら，その先にある臨床応用の追求は，今後も継続しなければ自然
美への到達は成し得ないだろう．

天然組織への挑戦が，今後も我々を奮い立たせてくれることを期待している．

Case 1

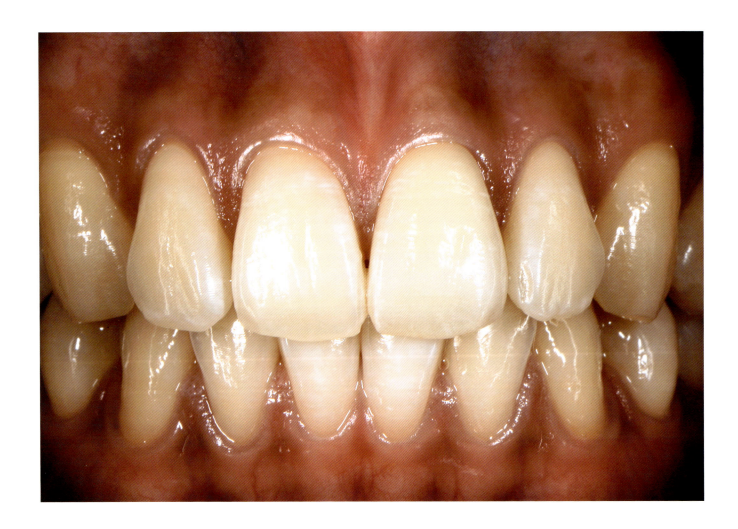

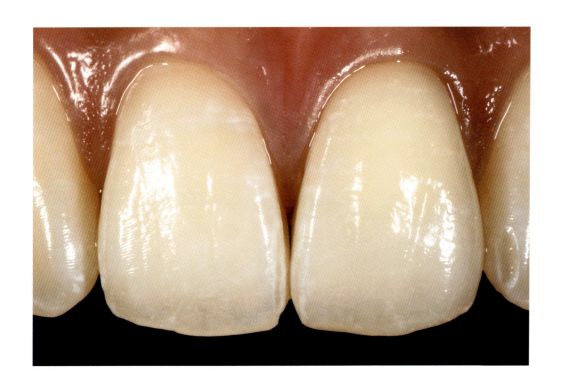

#9 IPS e.max Crown

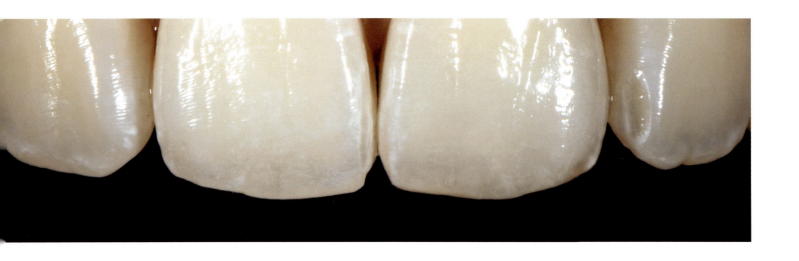

Fine Details : Is it just a decoration?

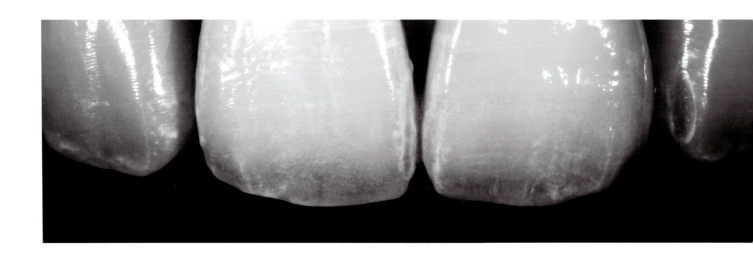

Case 2

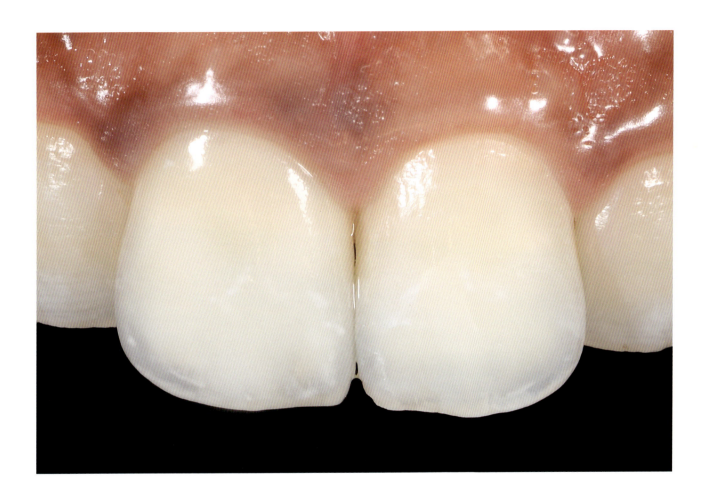

#8 IPS e.max Crown

Case 3

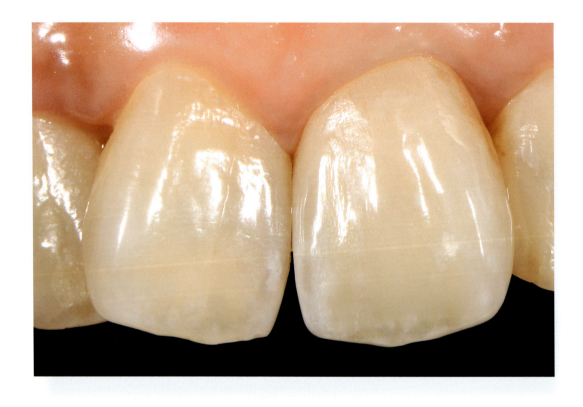

#9 IPS e.max Crown

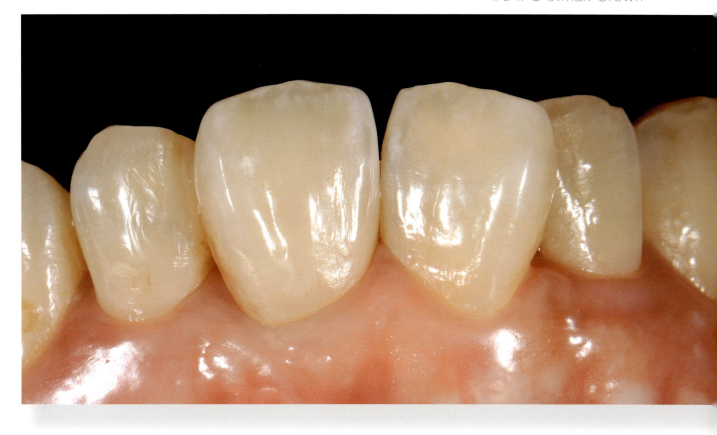

Case 4

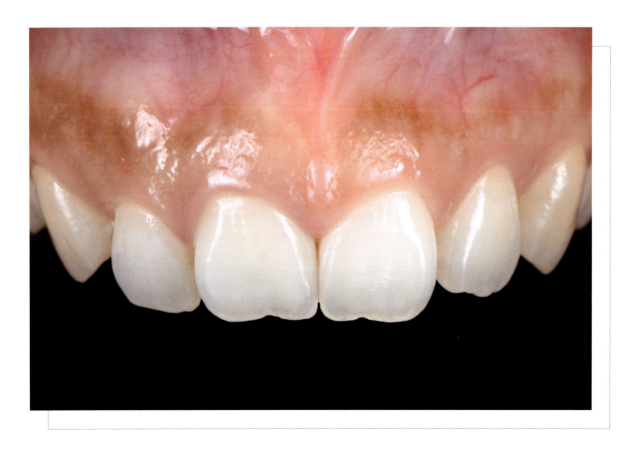

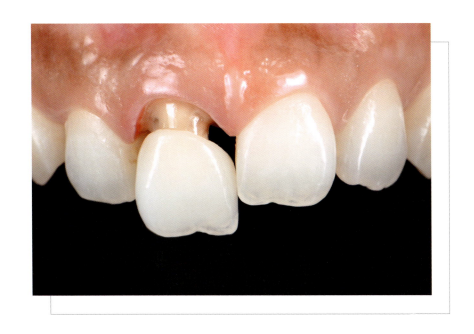

#8 IPS e.max Crown

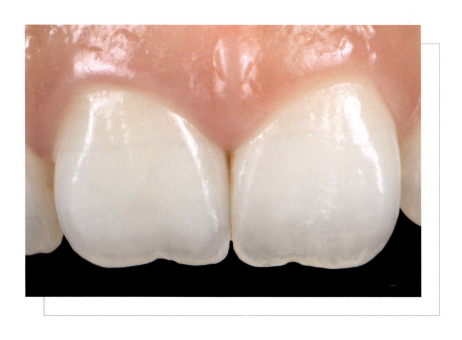

Case 5

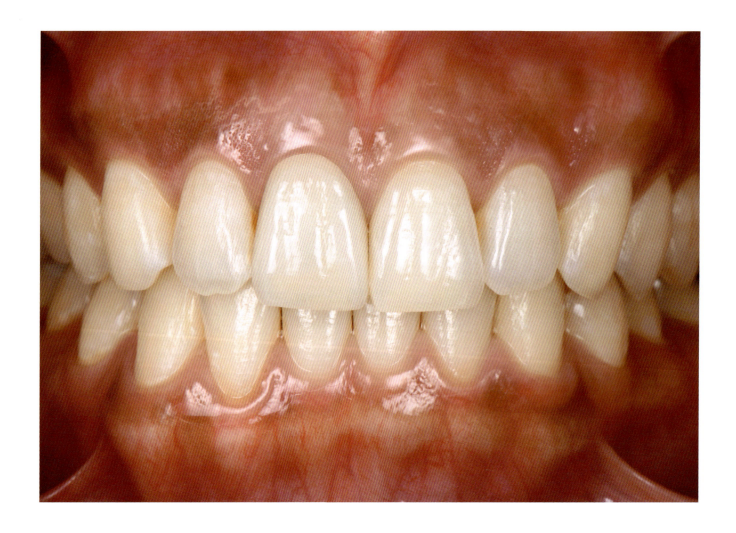

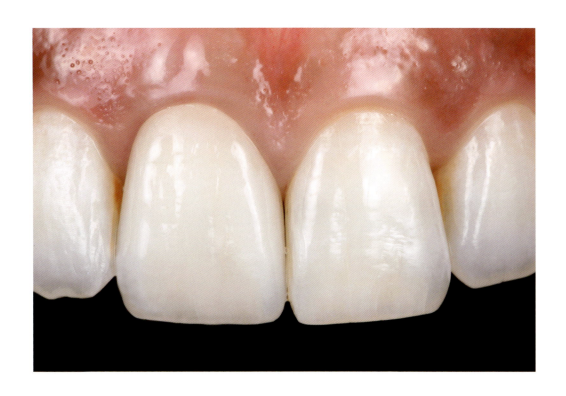

#8 IPS e.max Crown

Case 6

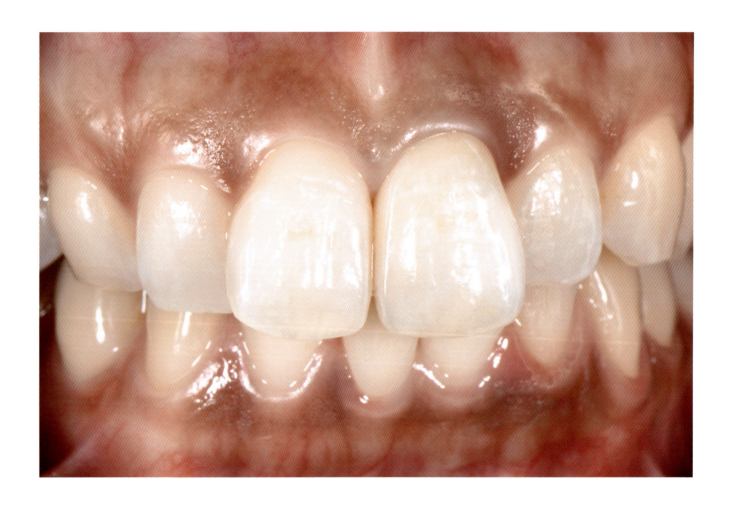

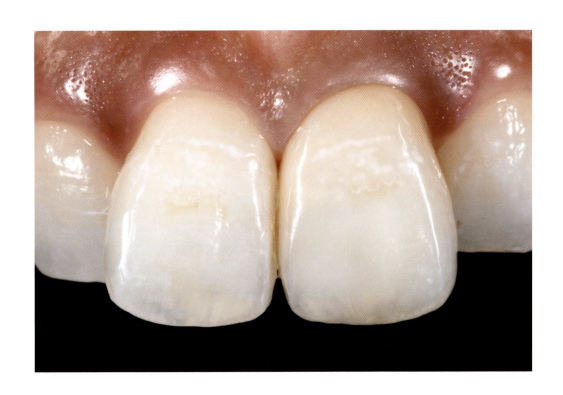

#9 IPS e.max Crown

Case 7

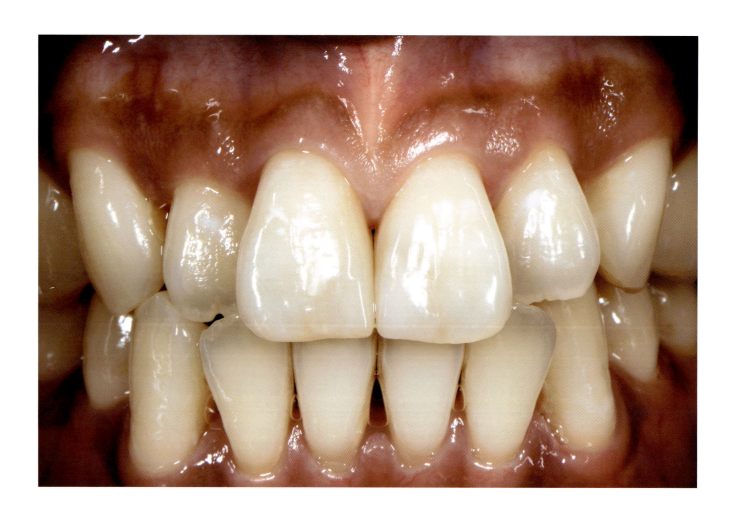

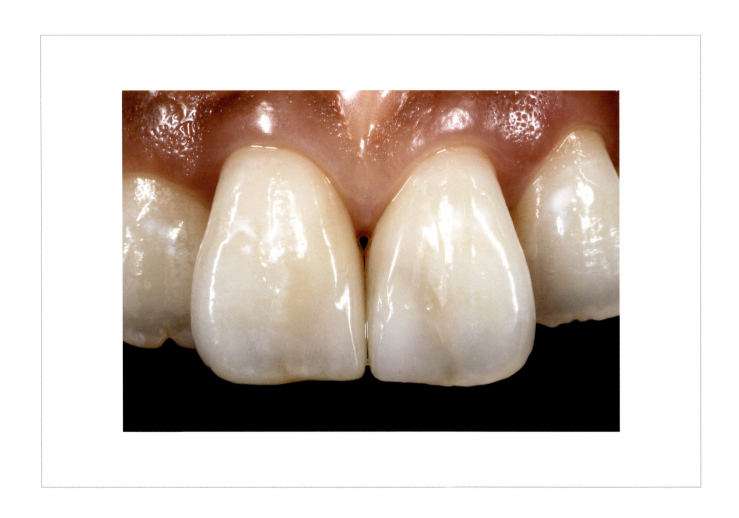

#8 IPS e.max Crown

Case 8

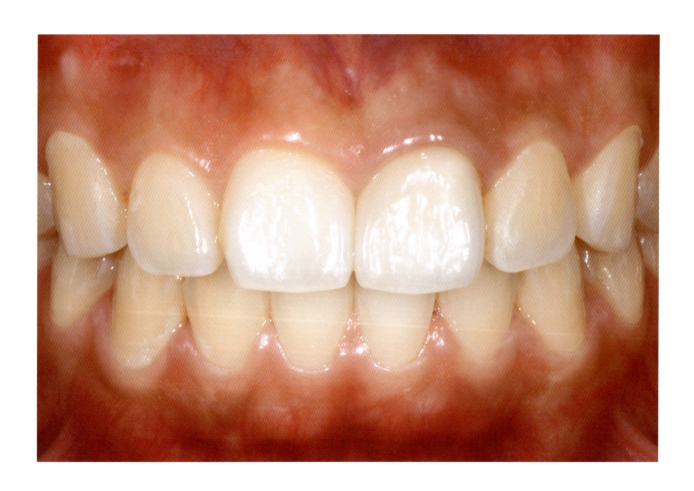

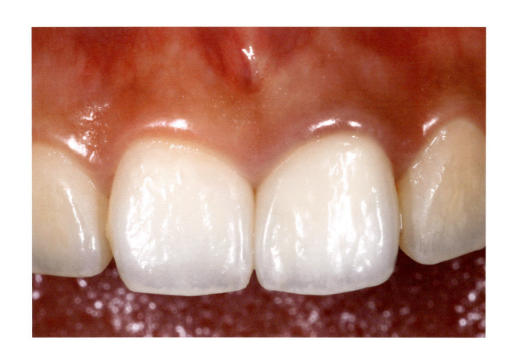

#9 IPS e.max Crown

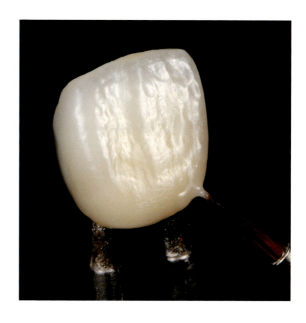

Case 9

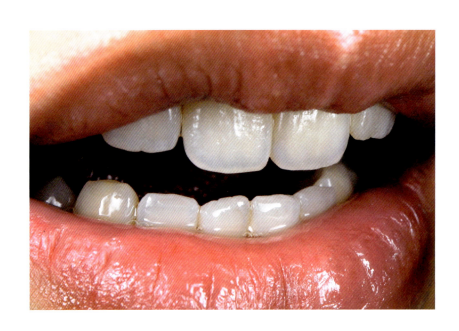

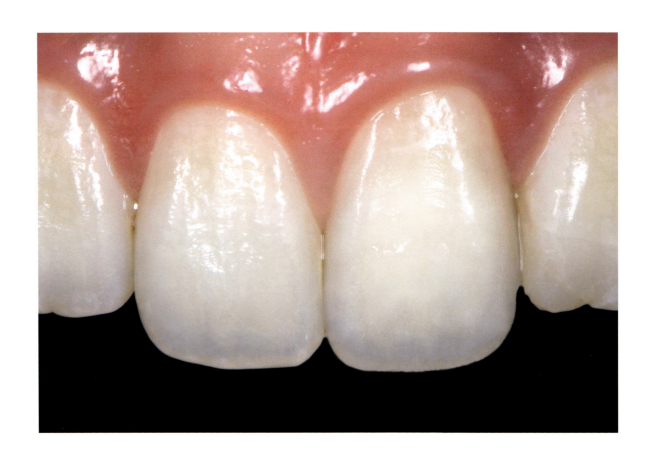

#9 IPS e.max Crown

Case 10

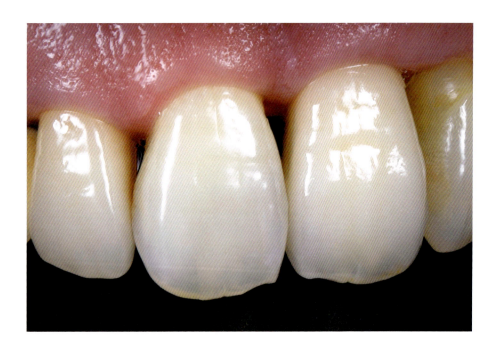

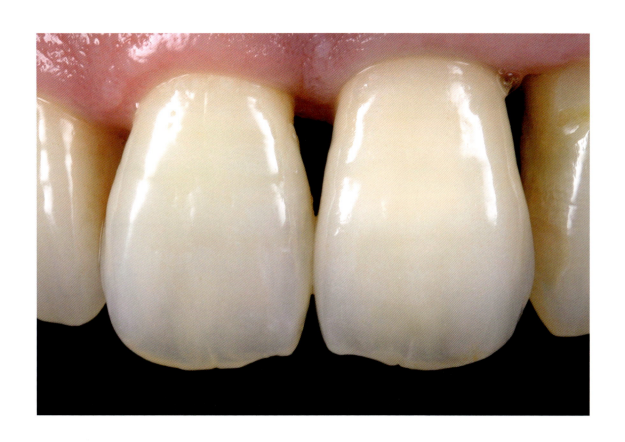

#9 IPS e.max Crown

Case 11

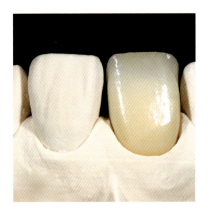
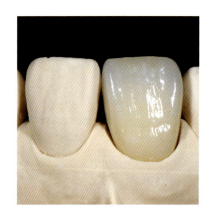
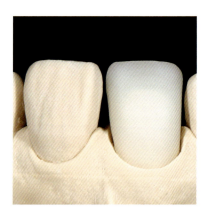

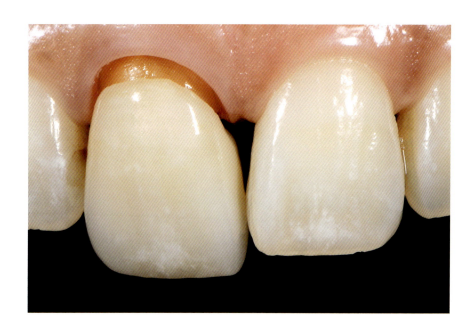

#8 IPS e.max Crown

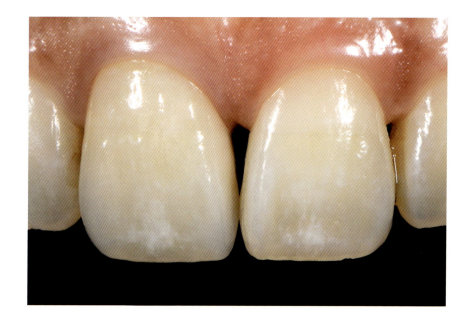

Case 12

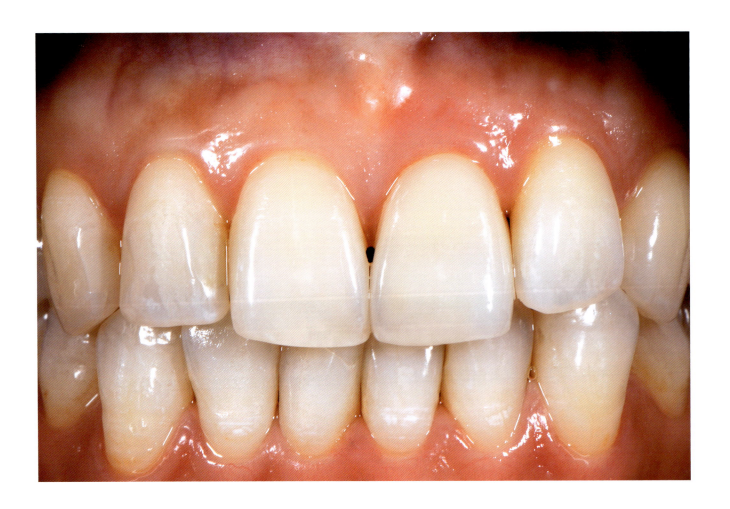

#9 IPS e.max Laminate Veneer

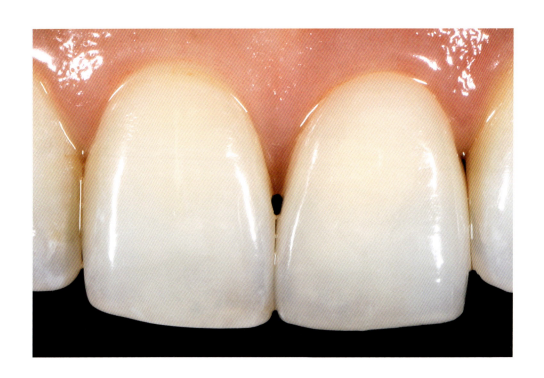
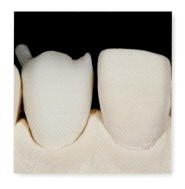
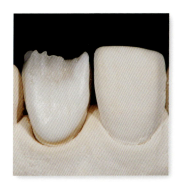
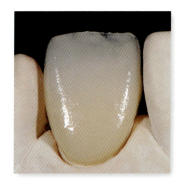

Case 13

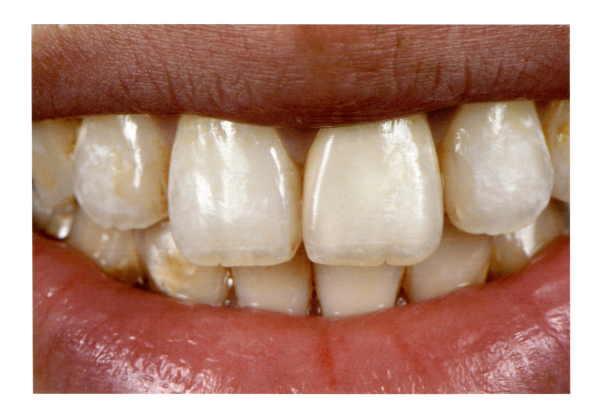

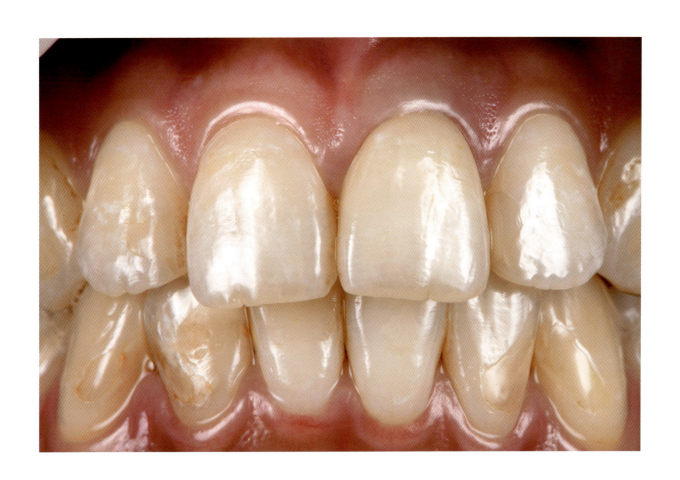

#9 IPS e.max Crown

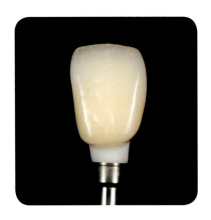

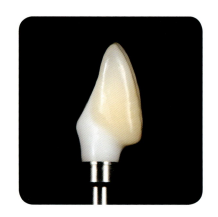

Case 14

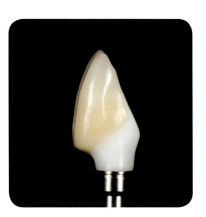

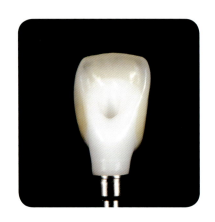

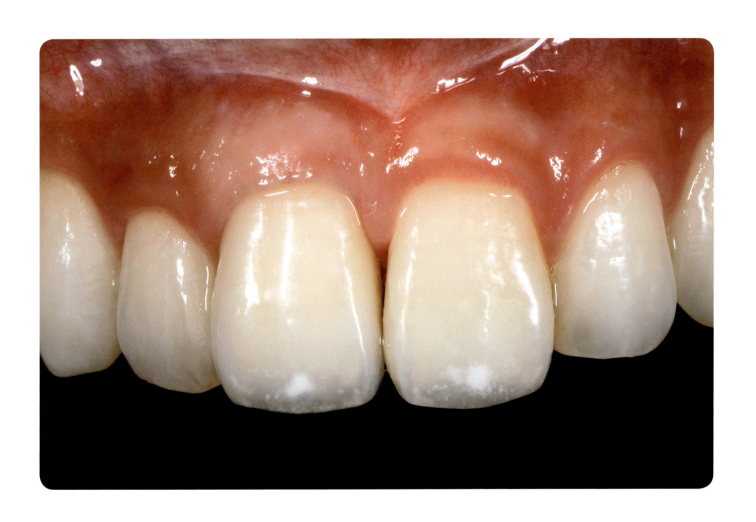

#8 IPS e.max Superstructure Solution

Case 15

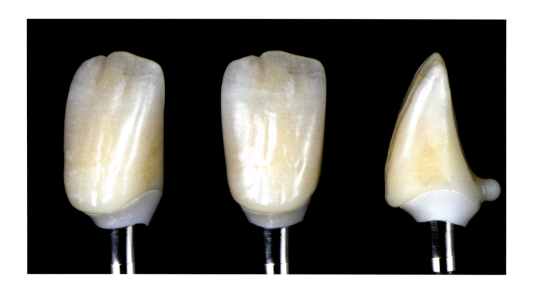

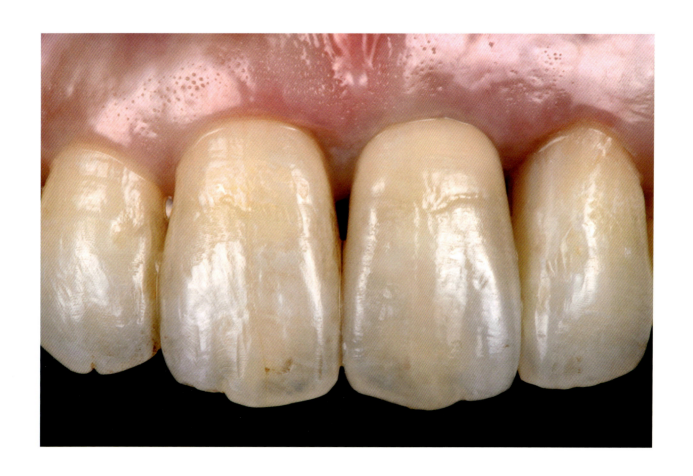

#9 IPS e.max Crown

Case 16

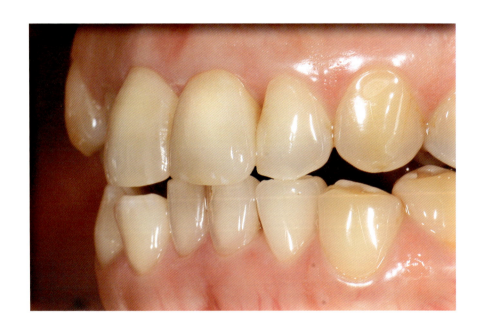

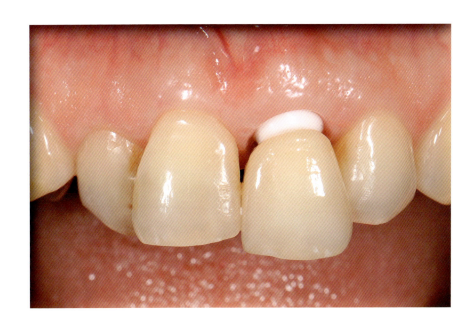

#9 IPS e.max Crown

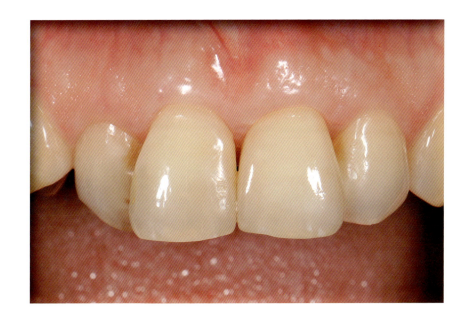

Case 17

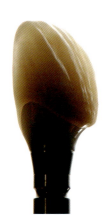 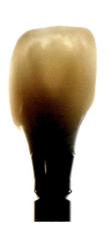 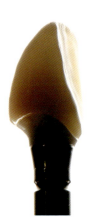

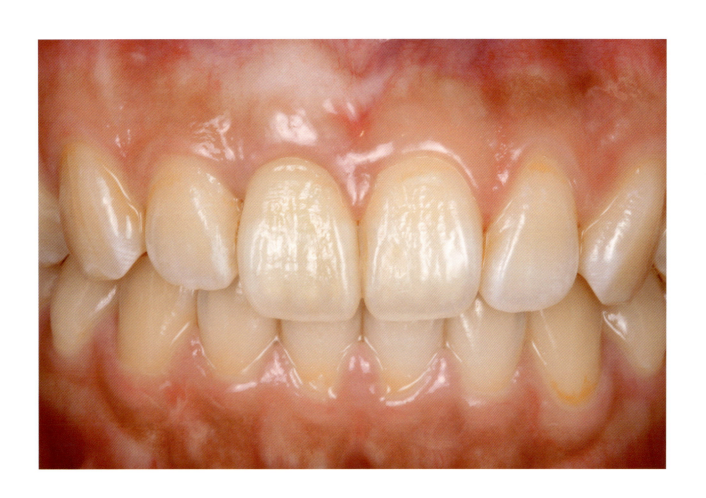

#8 IPS e.max Crown

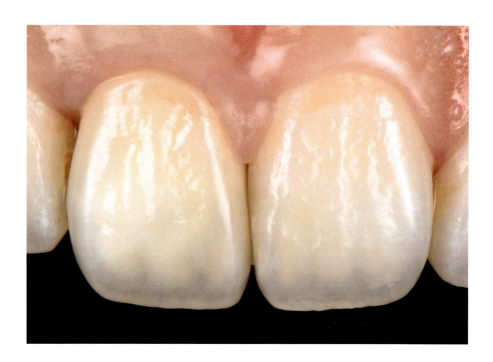

Surface Texture & Luster
It creates extremely fine details

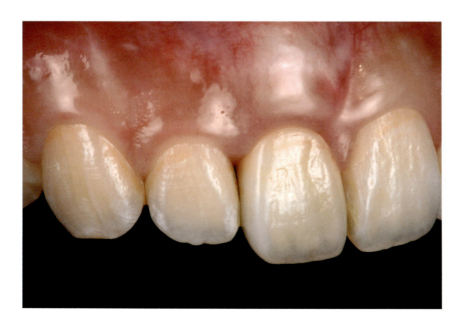
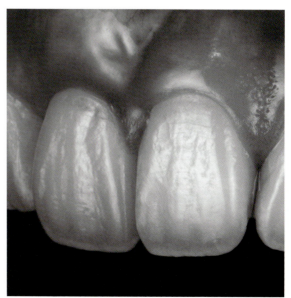

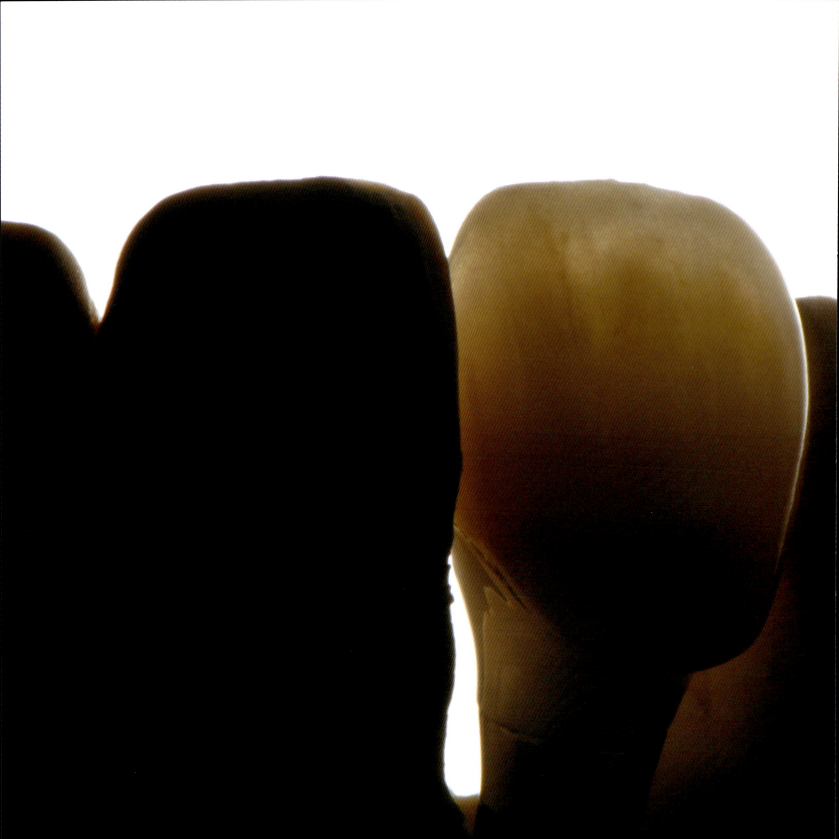

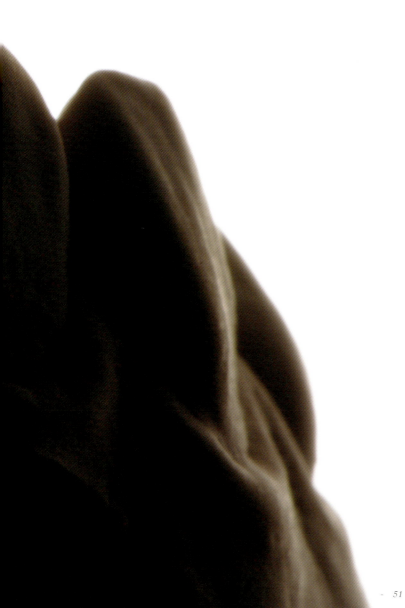

Light & Shade
Hybrid Superstructure

Case 18

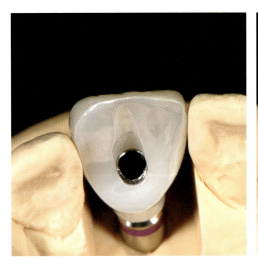
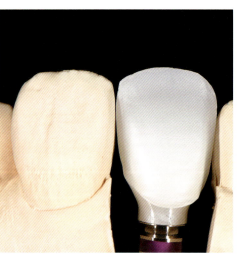
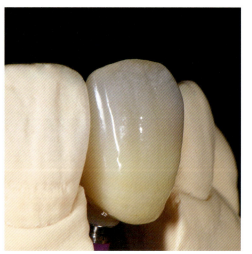

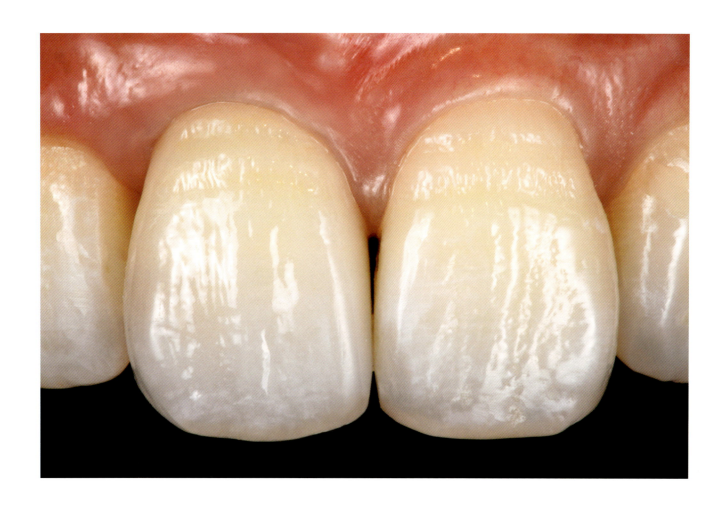

#8 IPS e.max Superstructure Solution

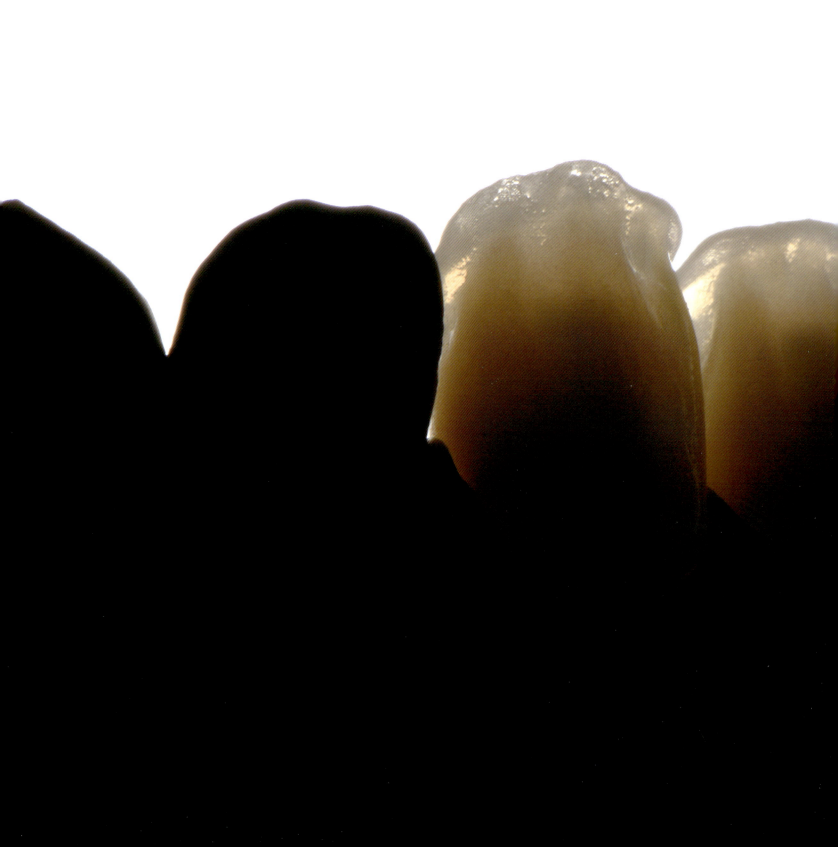

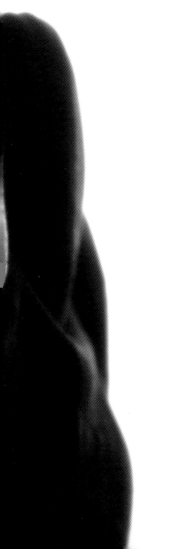

Part 2 : Individuality
Maxillary Central Incisors

「個性の表現」

上顎歯列全体に関わる中切歯の持つ存在感．それは，他にはない特有の個性を備えた部位であり，歯列のバランスを決定付ける多くの審美的要素が集約されている．

骨格と顔貌，歯列との調和，そして口唇とその動き．さらに，患者のコンプレックスにも配慮しながら，機能的かつ審美的な表現を心がけなければならない．

また，口唇を介してディスプレイされる歯は，切縁の適切な位置設定から始まり，唇側軸面形態と上部鼓形空隙のコントロールによって歯冠形態に個性を付与していく．ひいては，唇側歯冠部の遠心側の外形が歯列の形態やバランスに大きく影響を与えている．

歯冠形態の設計は，時に男性的に，そして女性的に．歯冠審美が与える客観的な印象を加味しながら，常にオリジナリティーを意識した個性を模索しなければならない．

Case 19

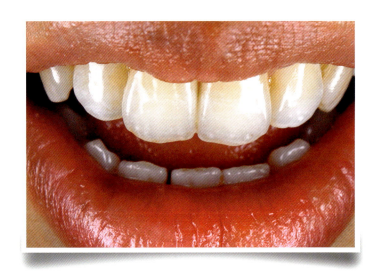

#8,9 IPS e.max Crown

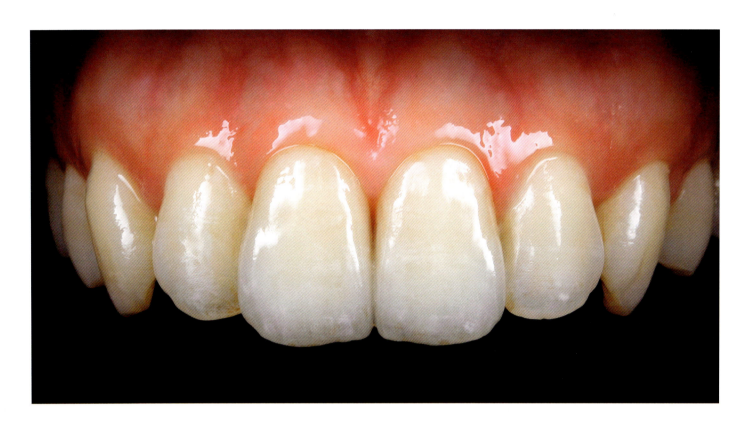
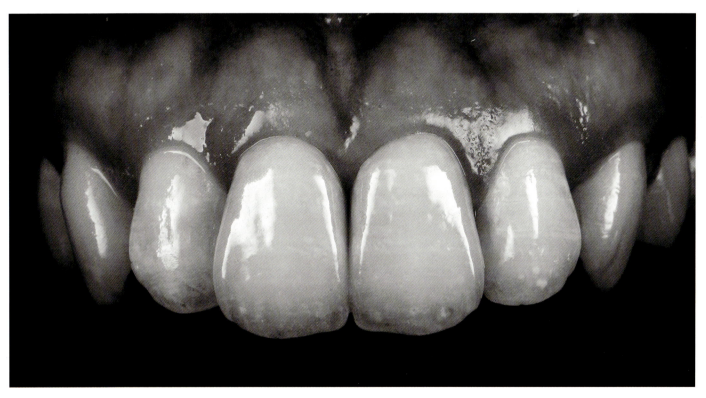

Case 20

#8,9 IPS e.max Crown

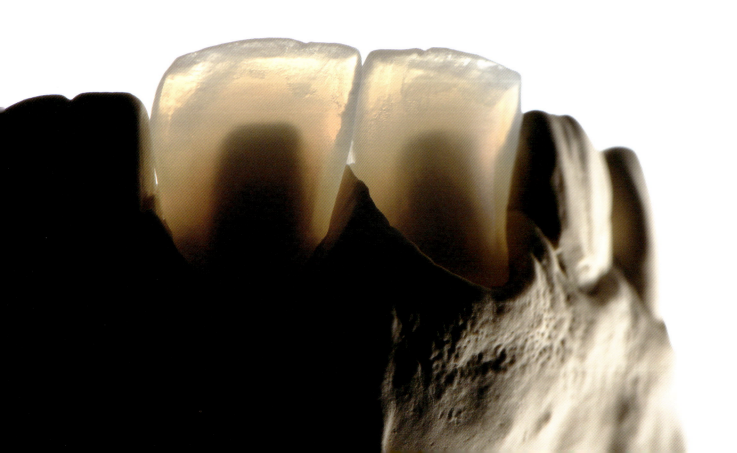

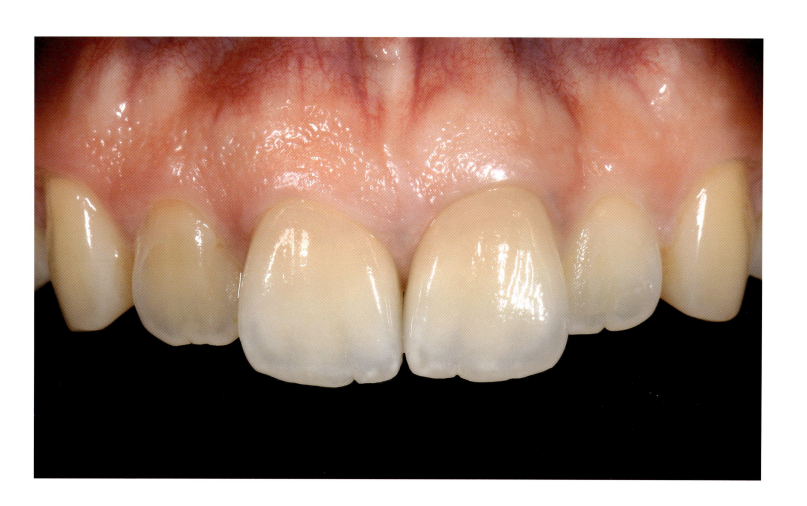
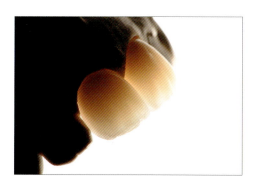
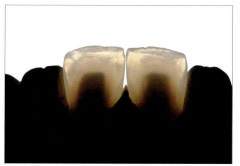
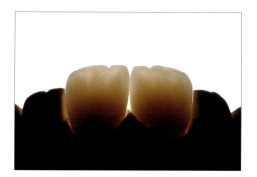

Case 21

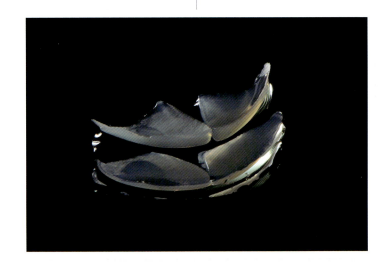

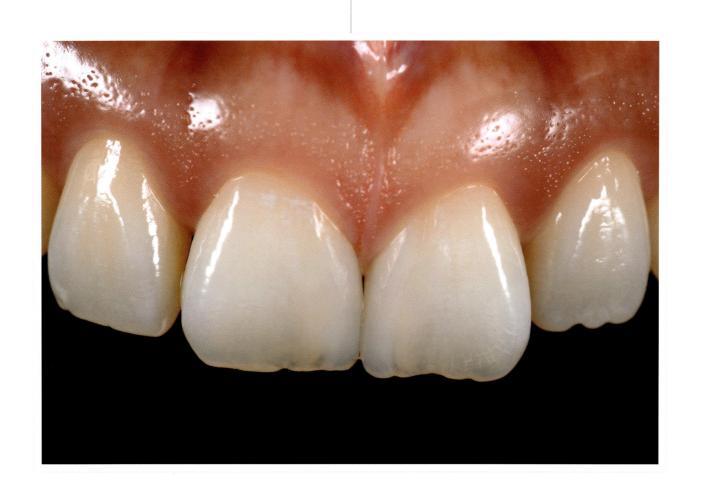

#8,9 IPS e.max Additional Laminate Veneer

Case 22

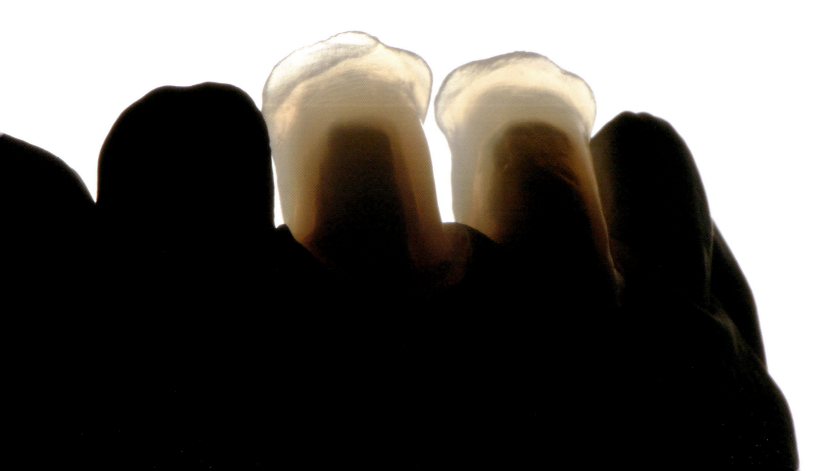

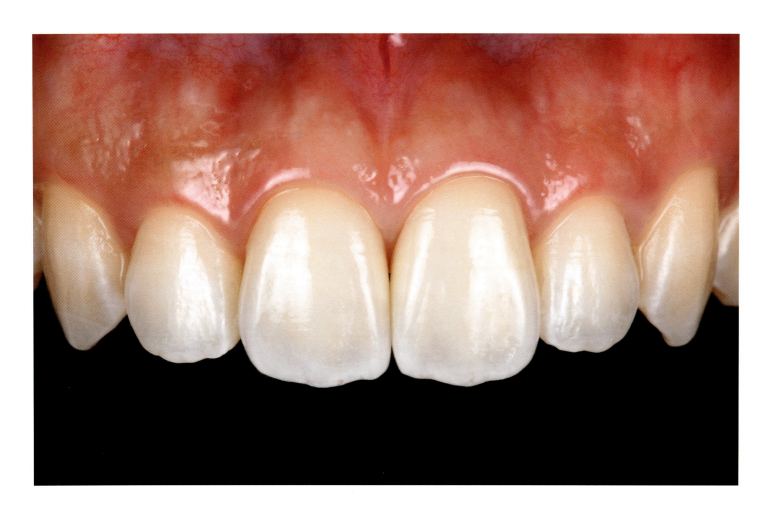

#8,9 IPS e.max Crown

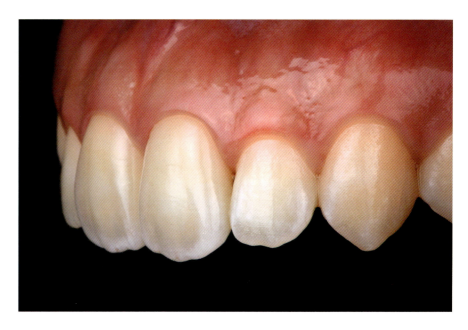

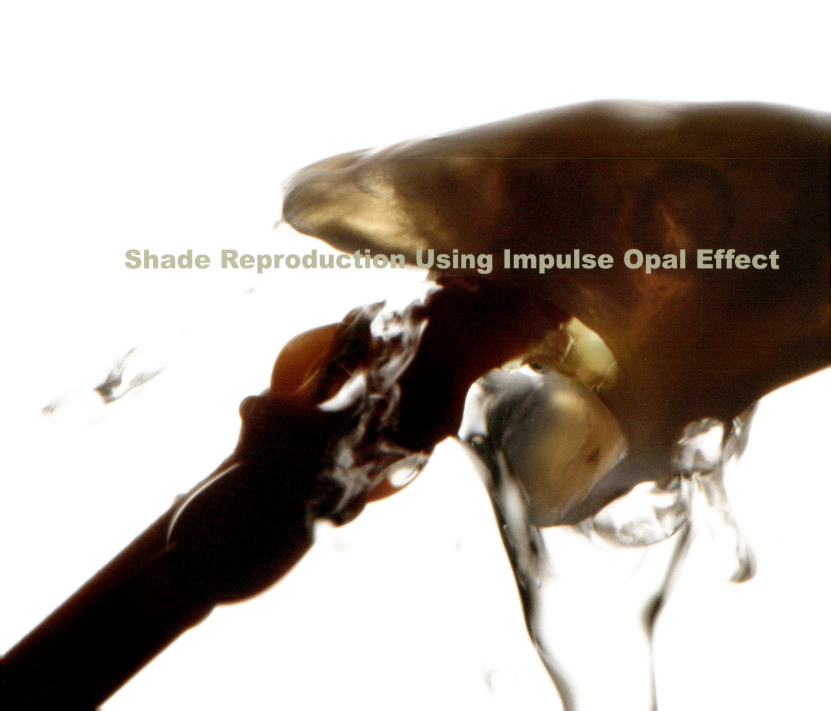
Shade Reproduction Using Impulse Opal Effect

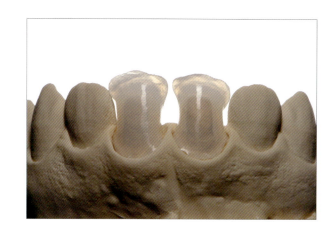
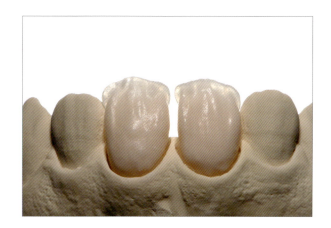

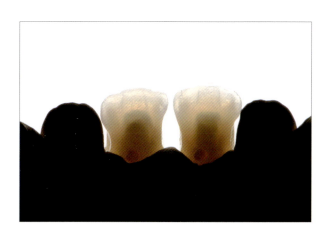

Case 23

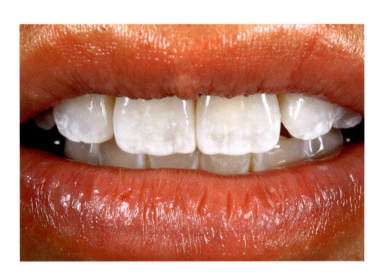

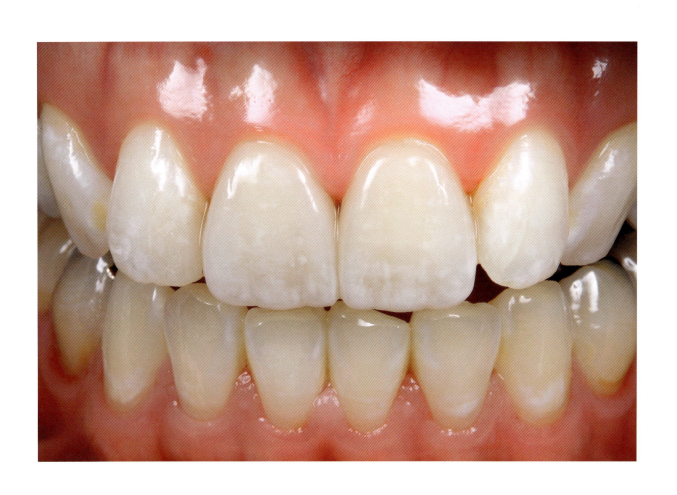

#8,9 IPS e.max Laminate Veneer

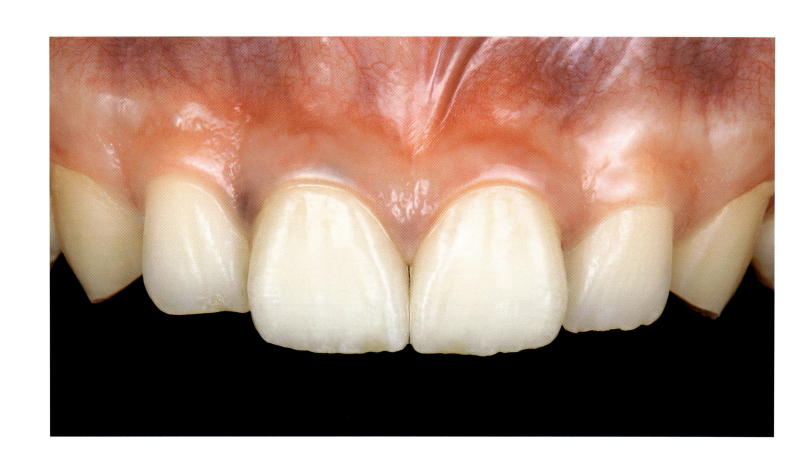

#8,9 IPS e.max Crown

Case 24

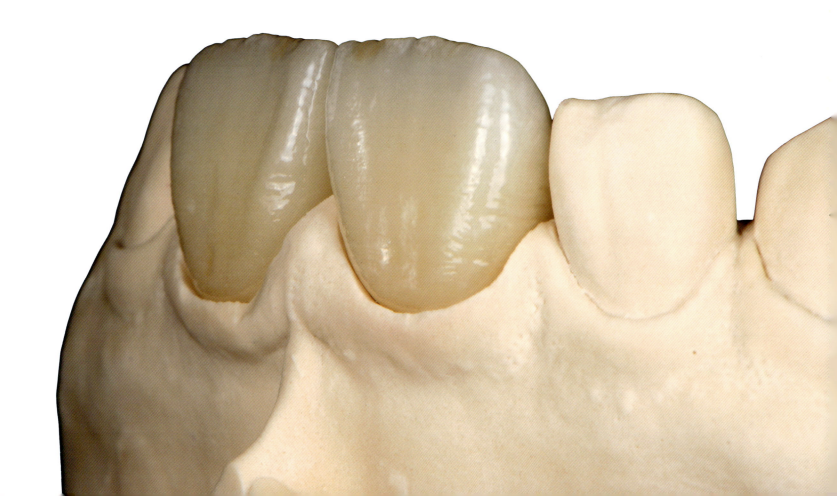

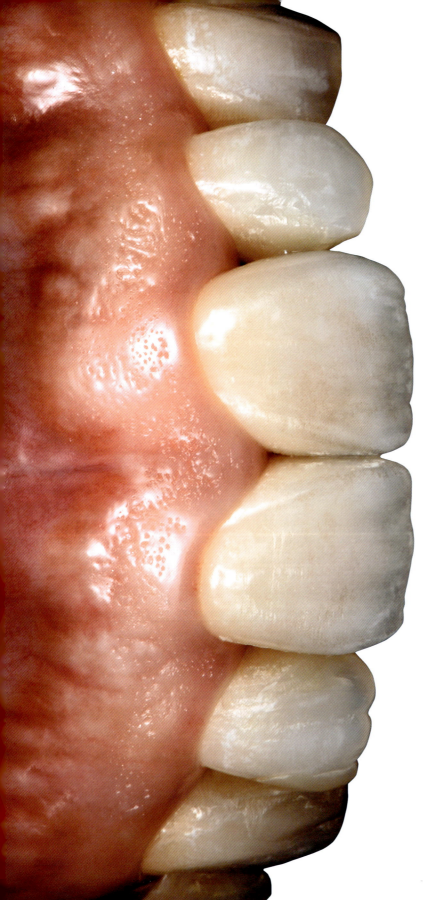

Case 25

#8,9 IPS e.max Crown

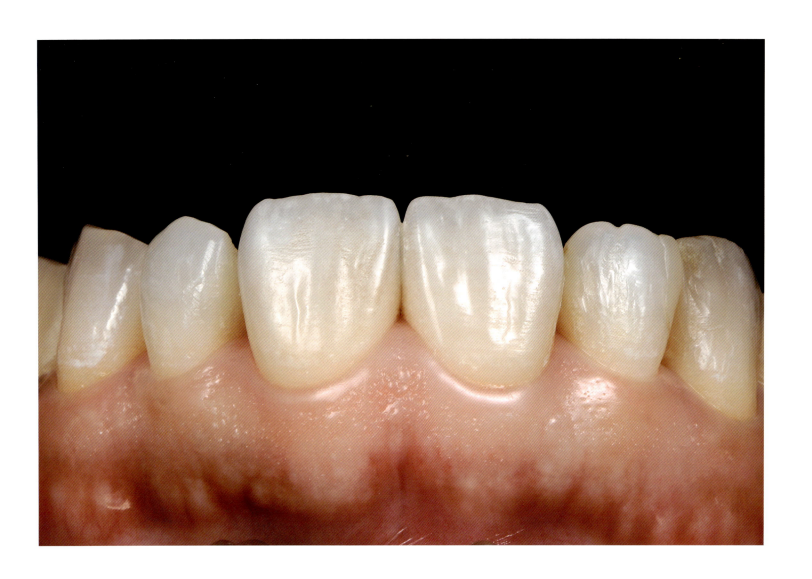

Case 26

Reproduction of Individuality

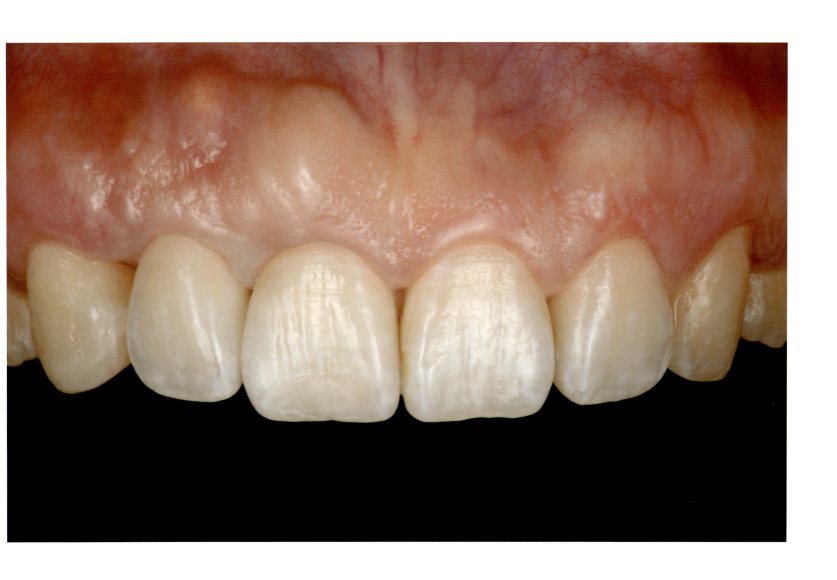

#7,8 IPS e.max Crown

Case 27

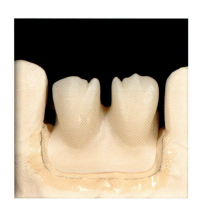
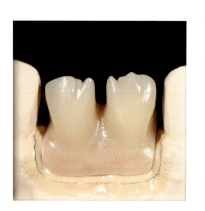
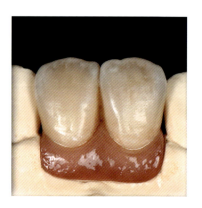

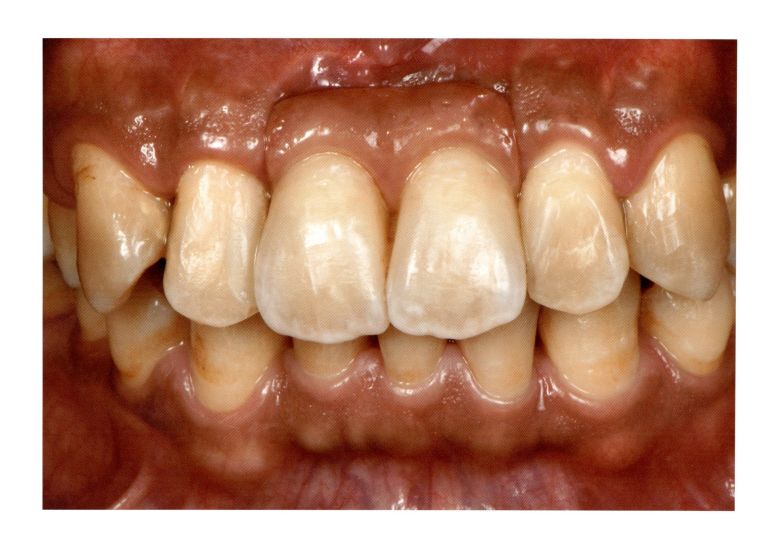

#8,9 IPS e.max Superstructure Solution

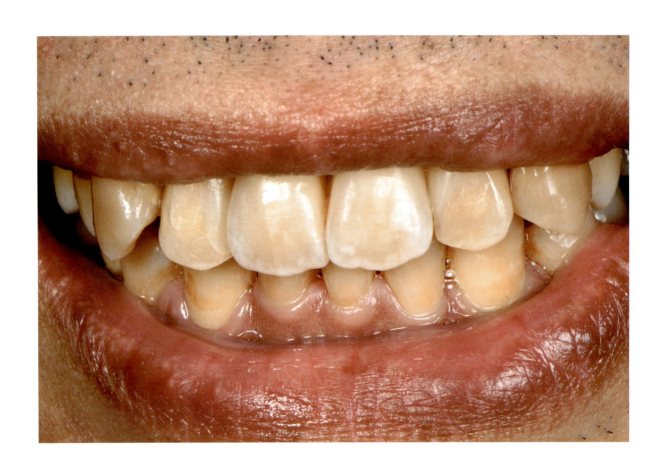

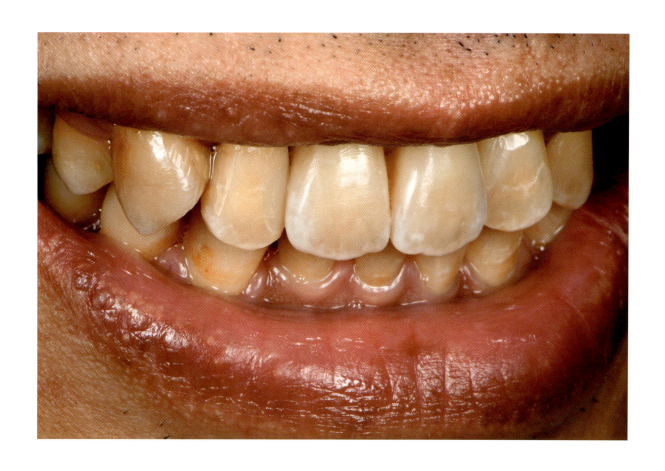

Harmony with Natural Dentition

IPS e.max
Superstructure Solution

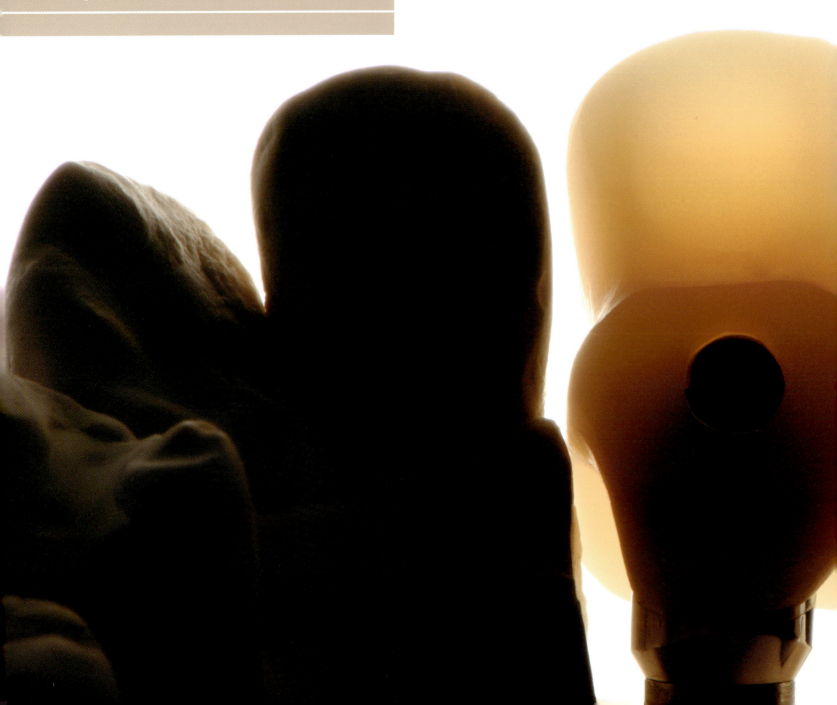

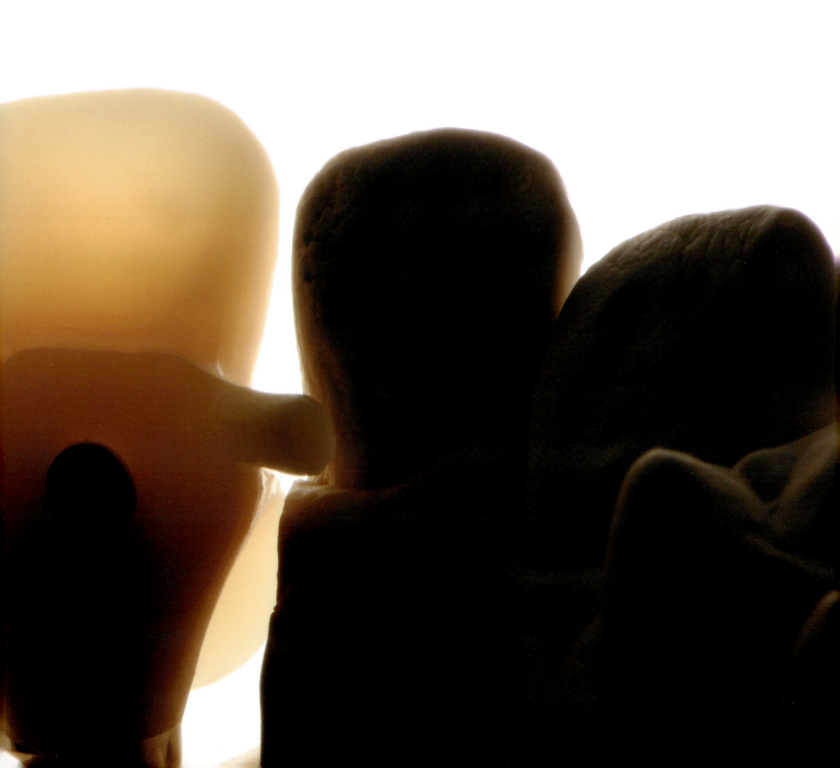

Case 28

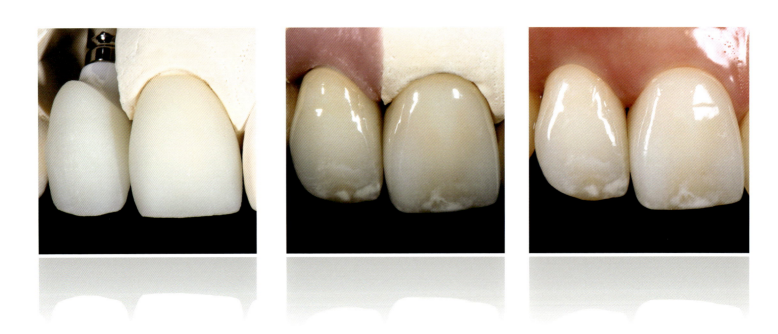

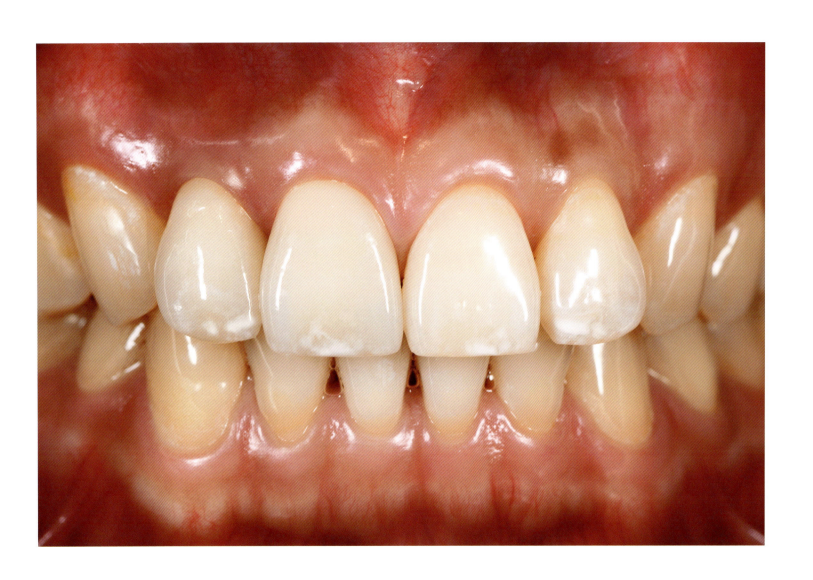

#7,8 IPS e.max Crown

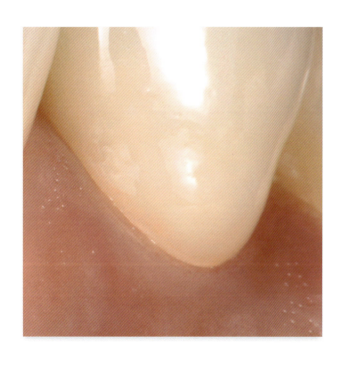
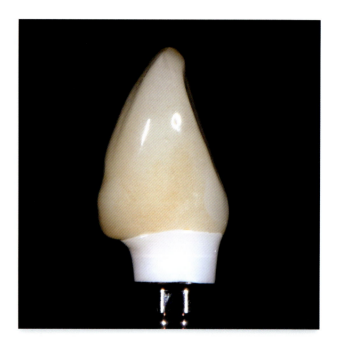

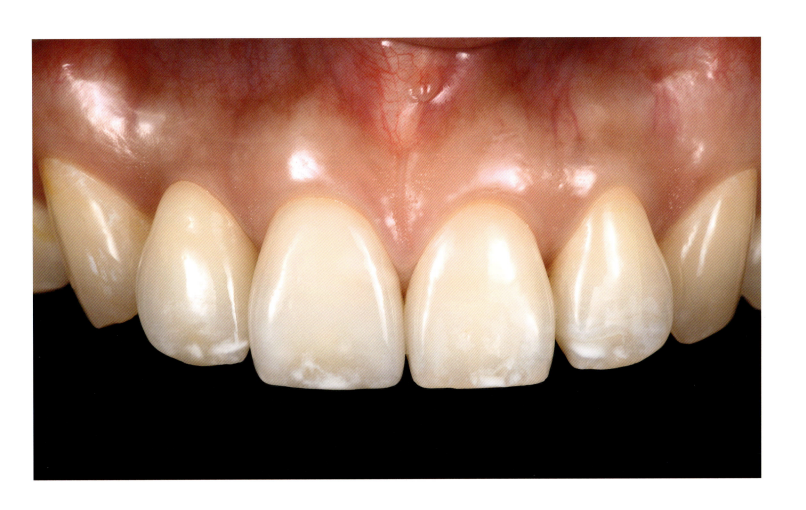

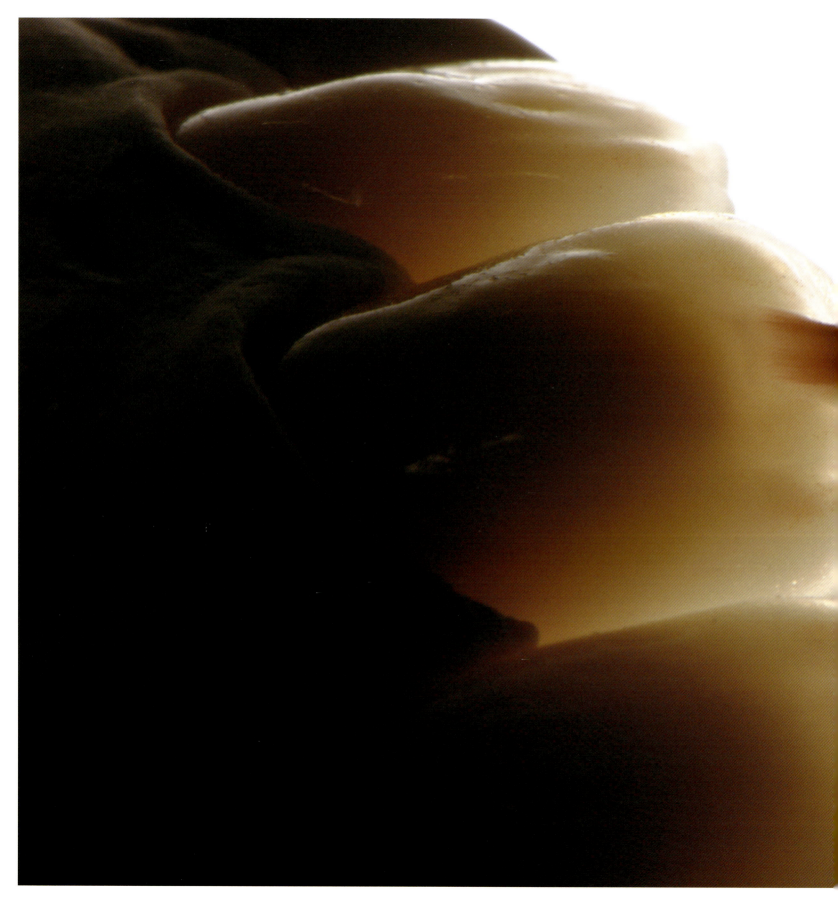

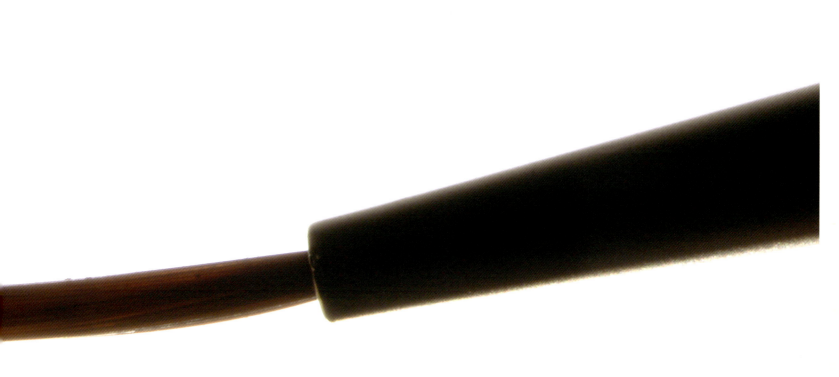

Part 3 : Harmony
between Esthetic and Function

「審美への調和」

前歯部修復治療において，その修復範囲が広がるにつれ機能的な配慮は大きくなる．特に，前歯群の機能の要となる犬歯に修復が及ぶかどうかによって修復の難易度は変わり，同様に歯の欠損や対合関係によっても審美回復に影響を及ぼす．

よって，補綴環境が整えられないような状況においては，何らかのかたちで補綴製作への妥協的な負担を増幅させてしまう．

そのため，審美の獲得には，根本となる機能的な問題を事前に解決しておく必要があり，外科処置や矯正治療などを補綴前処置として効果的に組み込まなければならない場合が多い．

これは，同一の治療ゴールを描いた歯科医師との強い連携が治療結果に大きく反映されるということである．

問題を見極め，機能美を回復させることが審美獲得への第一歩となる．
機能的な釣り合いの取れた歯列にこそ自然美は存在しているのかもしれない．

Case 29

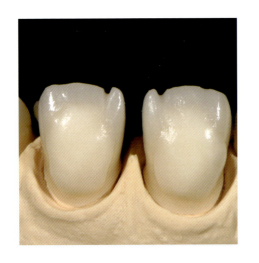
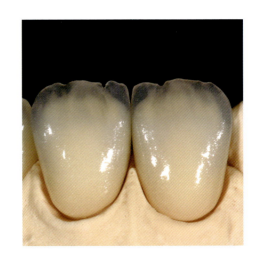
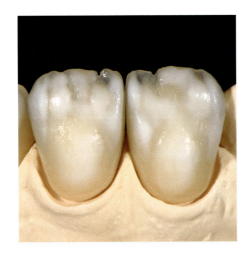
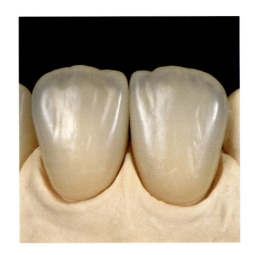

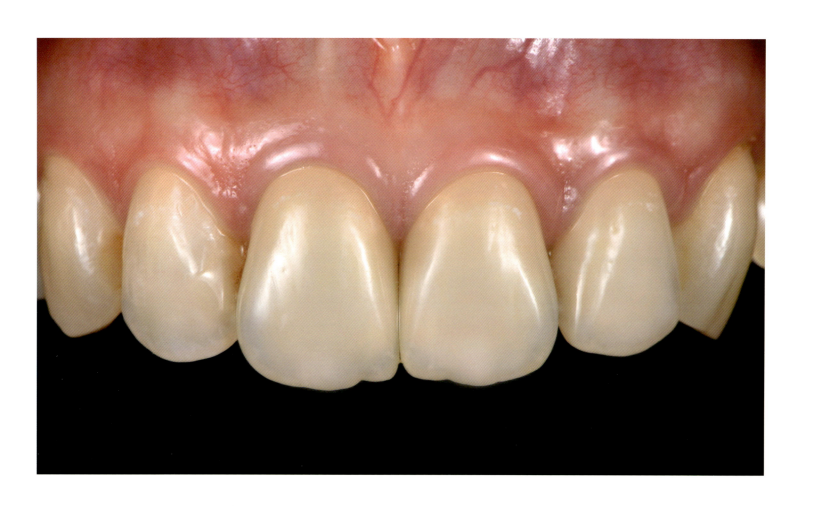

#8-10 IPS e.max Zirconia Crown

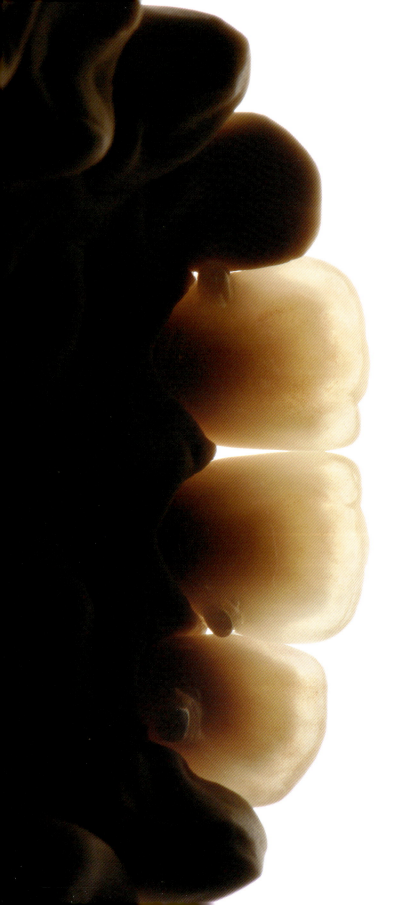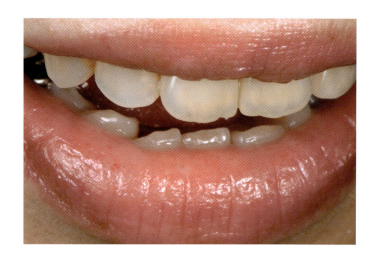

with Lips

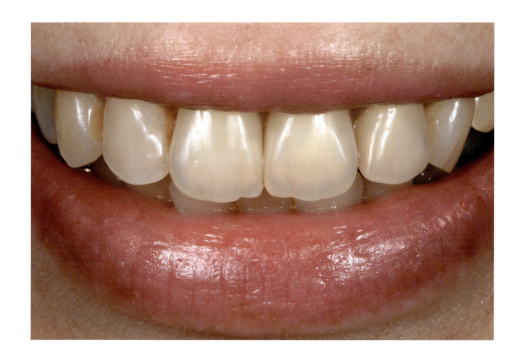

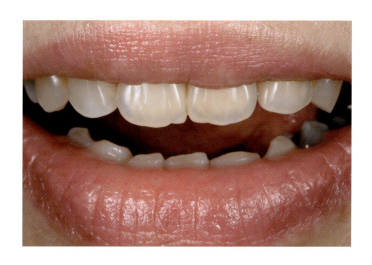

Case 30

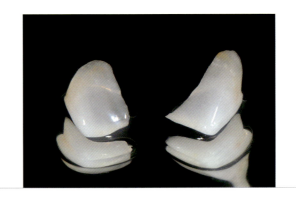

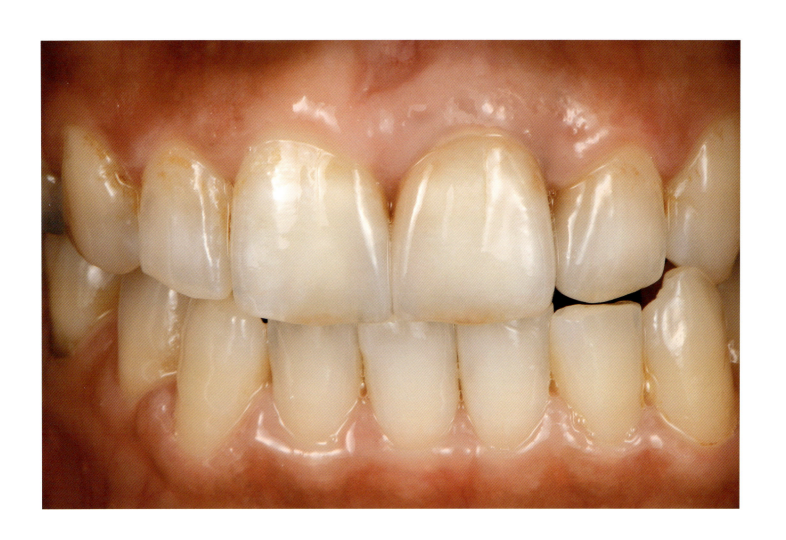

#8,10 IPS e.max Additional Laminate Veneer & #9 IPS e.max Crown

Case 31

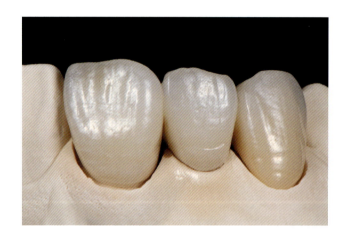

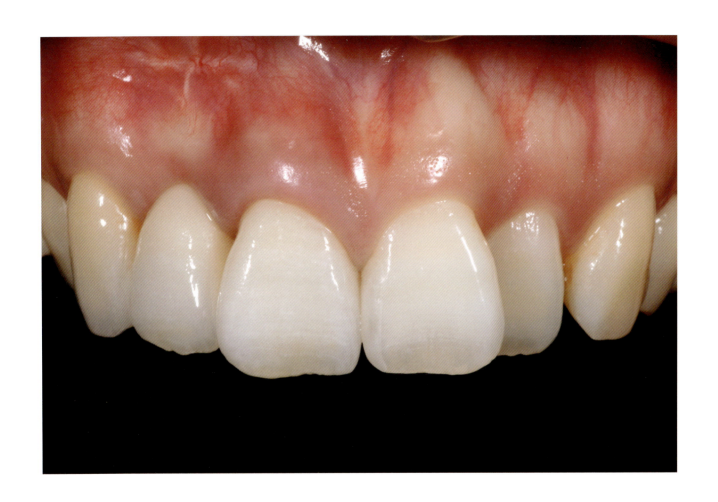

#6-8 IPS e.max Three Unit Bridge

Case 32

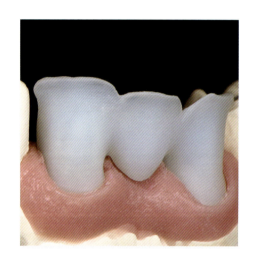
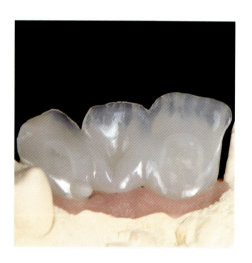

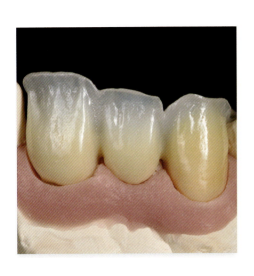
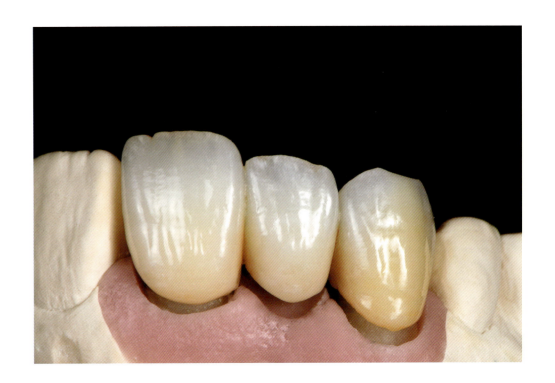

#6-8 IPS e.max Three Unit Bridge

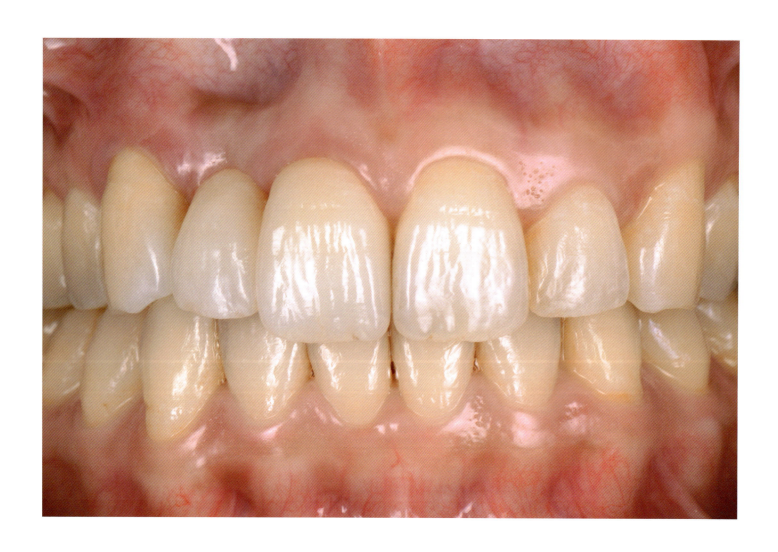

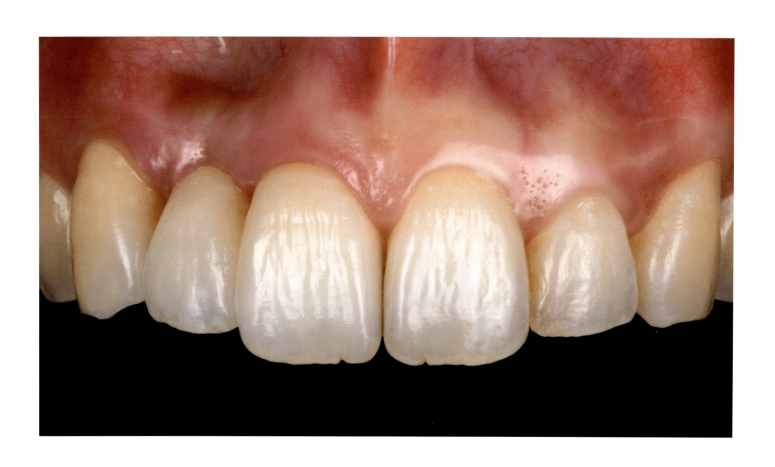

Case 33

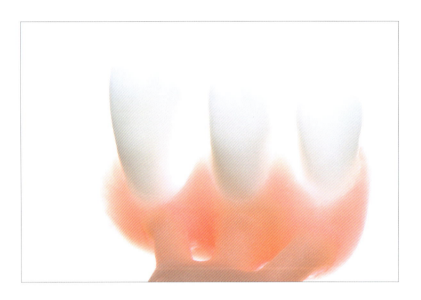

Adhesive Implant Superstructure Design

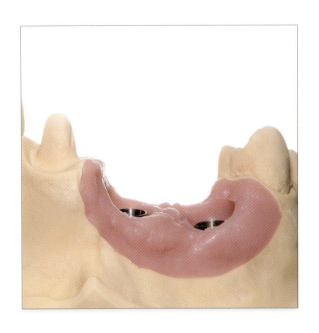
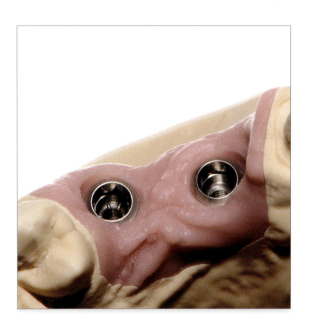
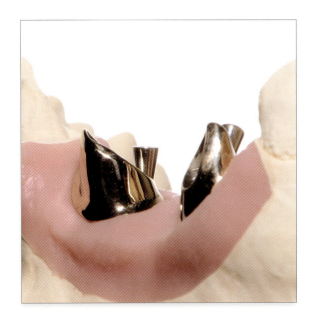
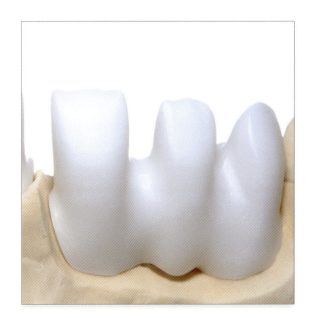

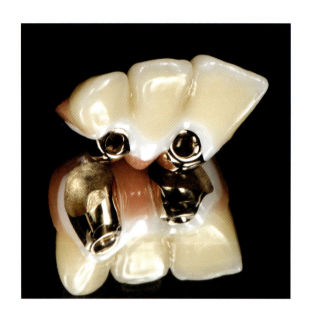 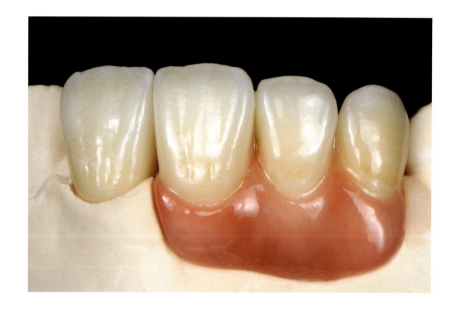

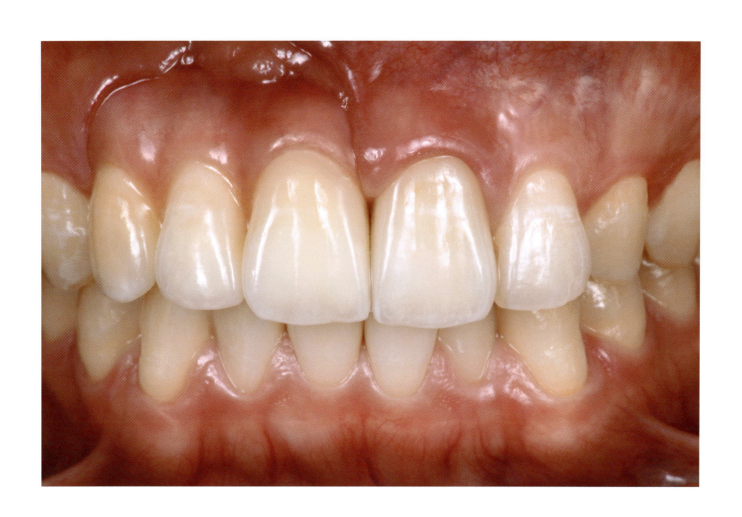

#6-8 IPS e.max Superstructure Solution

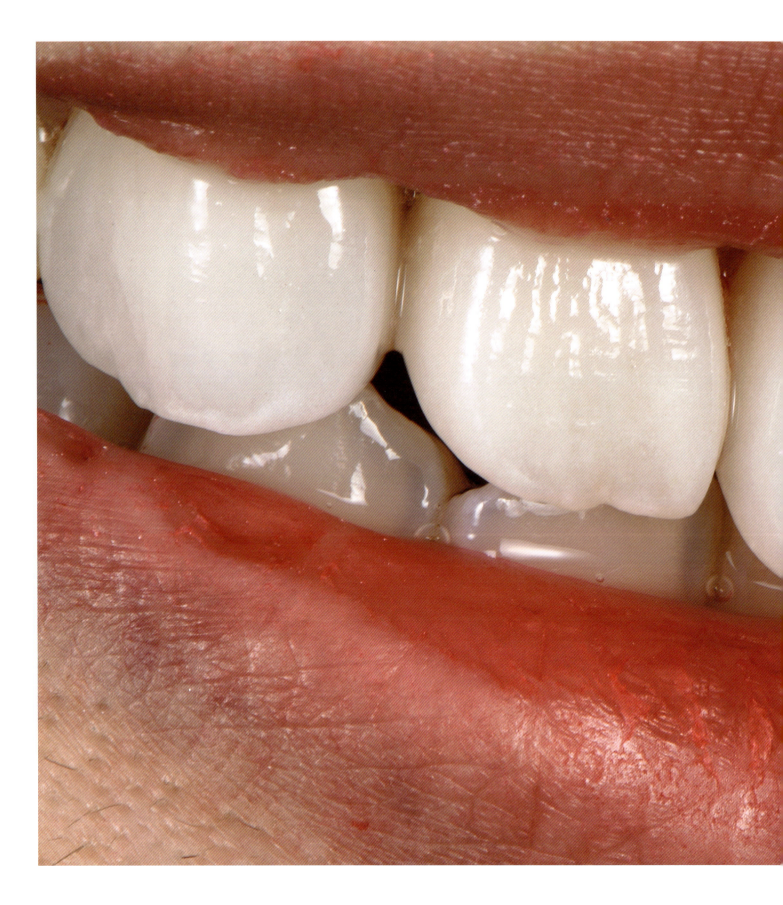

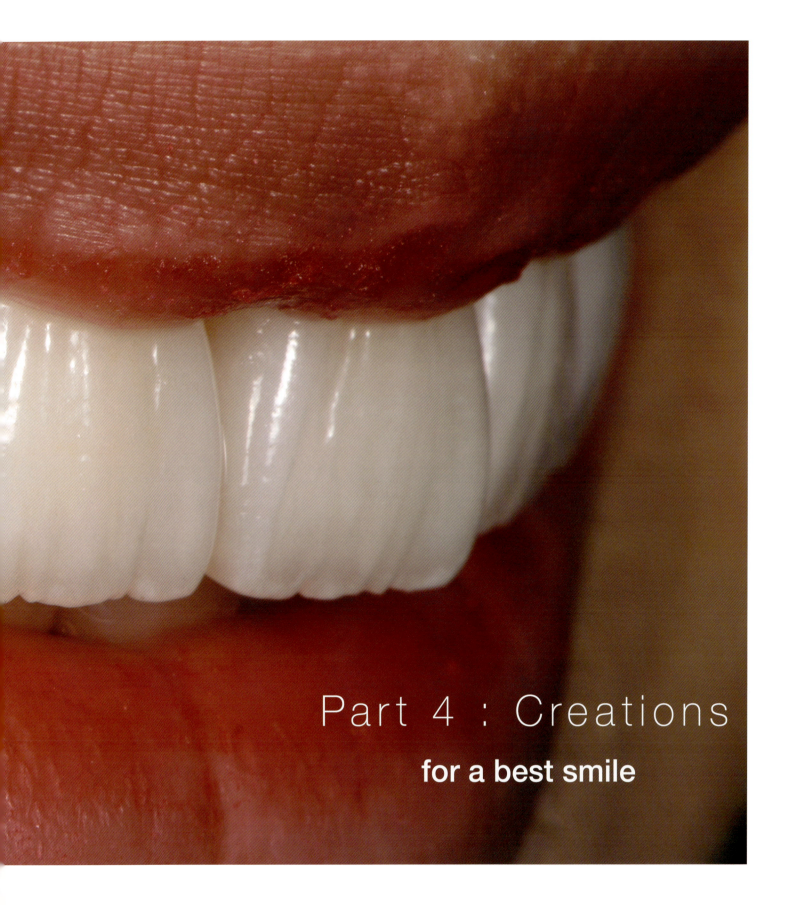

Part 4 : Creations
for a best smile

「Smile Design」

Smile Design，それは審美修復治療が迎える最終のゴールイメージである．
解剖学に沿った一歯単位の形態回復から，個性を交えた絶妙な配列表現を施し，口唇そして顔貌とのトータル的なバランスを図っていく．
それは，時に患者の性格やライフスタイル，容姿にも配慮しながら患者の持つ個性を最大限に引き出すことが重要だ．
そして，そこに加わるのが色調表現である．
ここでは，患者の持つ理想的な欲求が優先されることも少なくはないが，女性が行うメイクアップのように，肌の持つ色味との調和を考慮したり年齢等も踏まえたりしなければならない．

美しい歯列が与える印象は患者の心を高揚させ，ひいては私生活においても大きな充実感をもたらすだろう．
それはまさに，人の手によって創造された人工物が理想美を叶える瞬間となる．

喜びに満ちたその瞬間に立ち会えることは，作り手にとってこの上ない喜びとなる．

Case 34

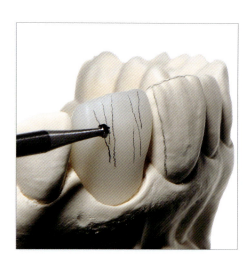

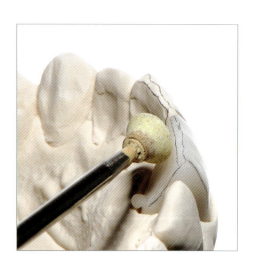

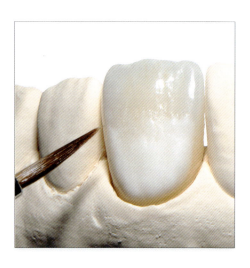

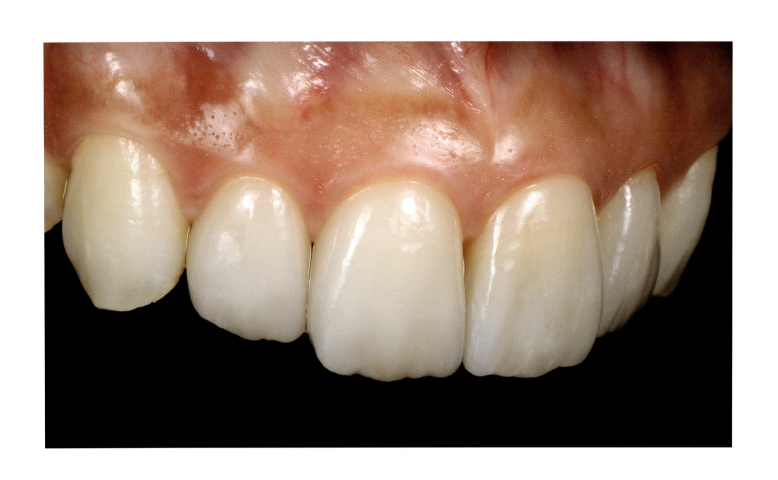

#7,8,10 IPS e.max Laminate Veneer & #9 IPS e.max Crown

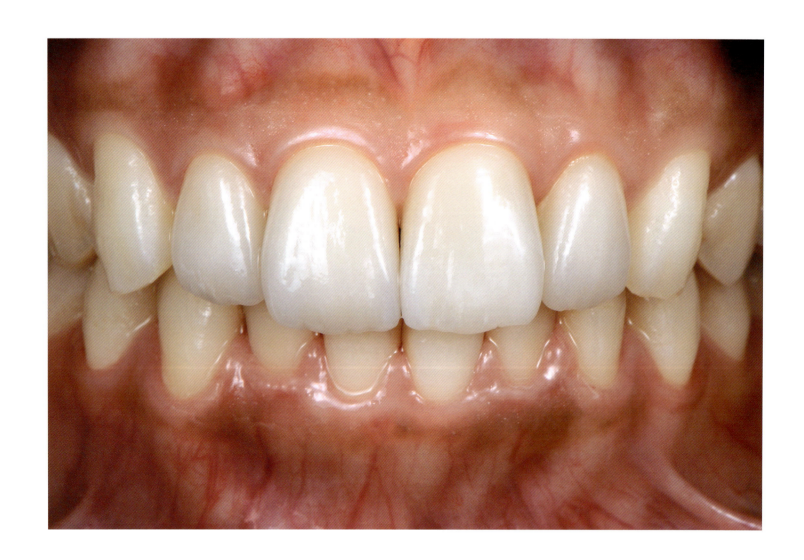

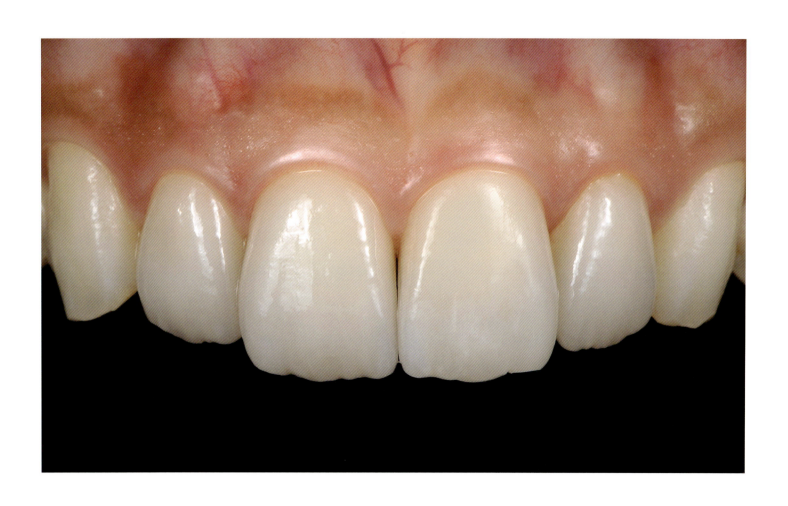

Case 35

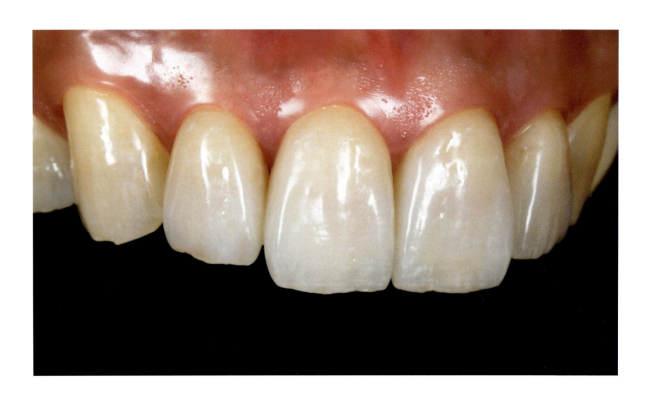

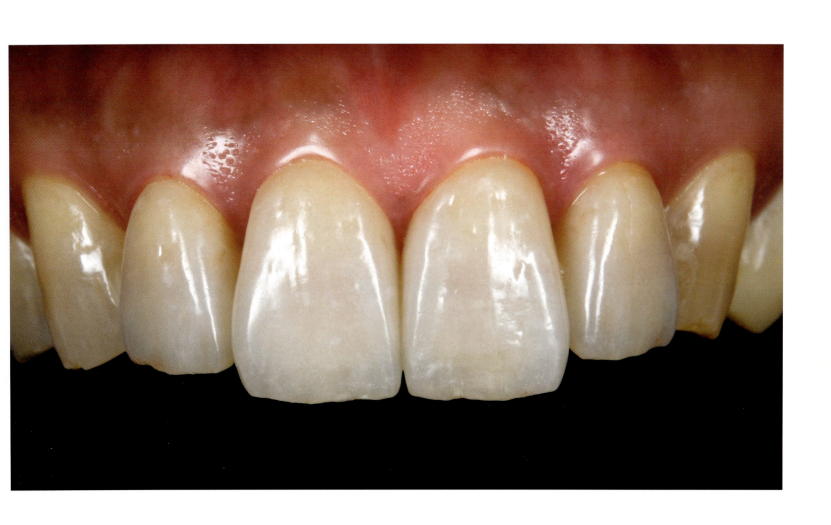

#7-10 IPS e.max Crown

Case 36

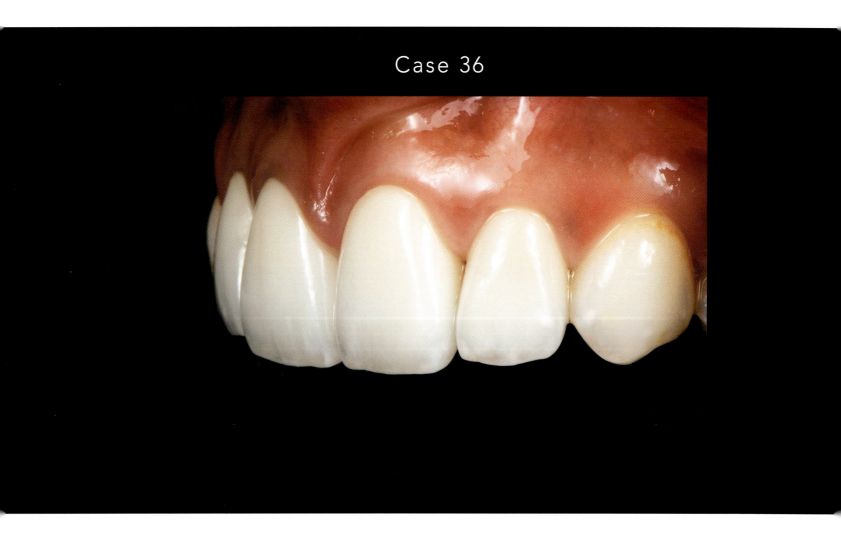

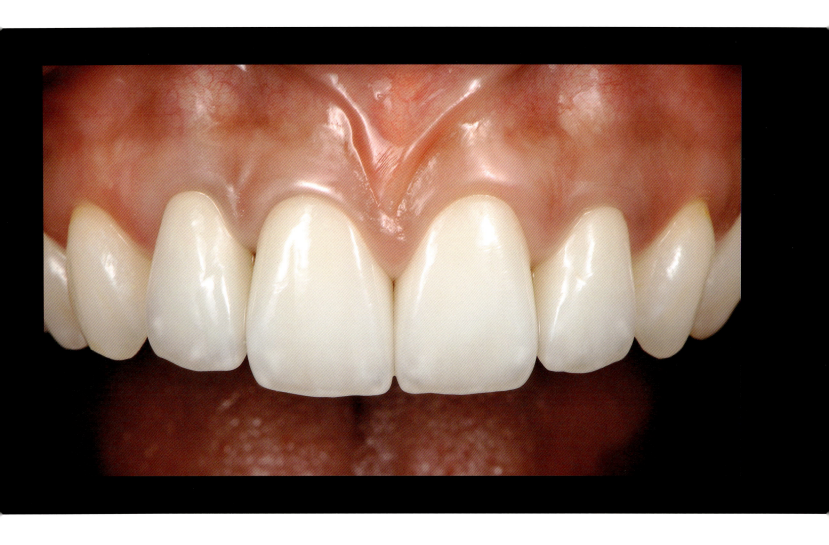

#7-10 IPS e.max Crown

Case 37

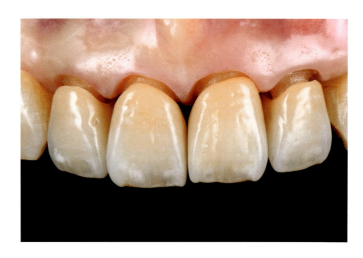

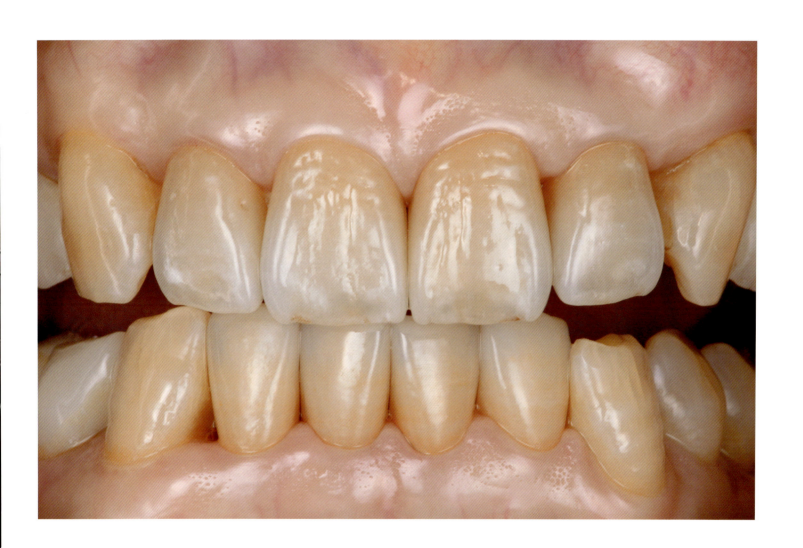

#7-10 IPS e.max Crown

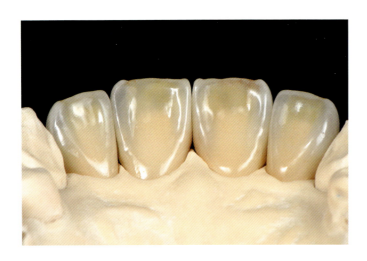

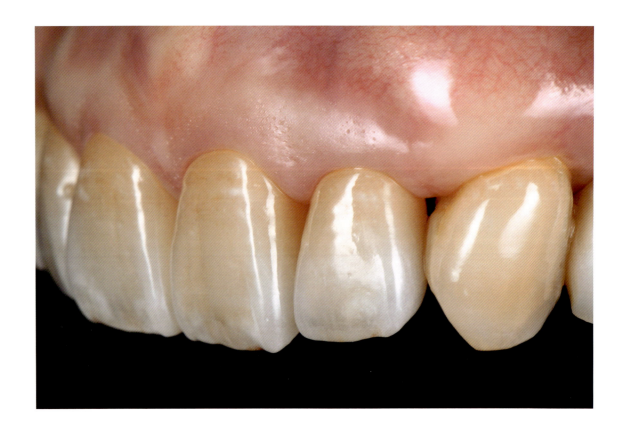

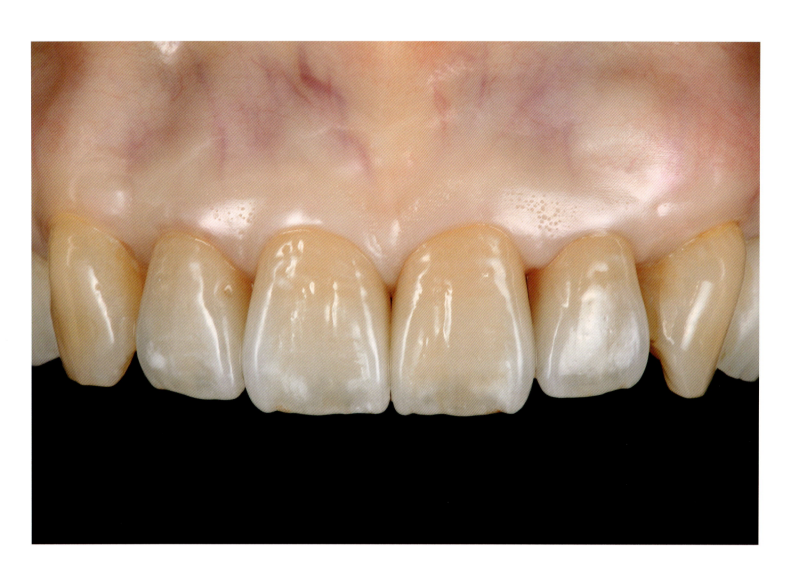

Case 38

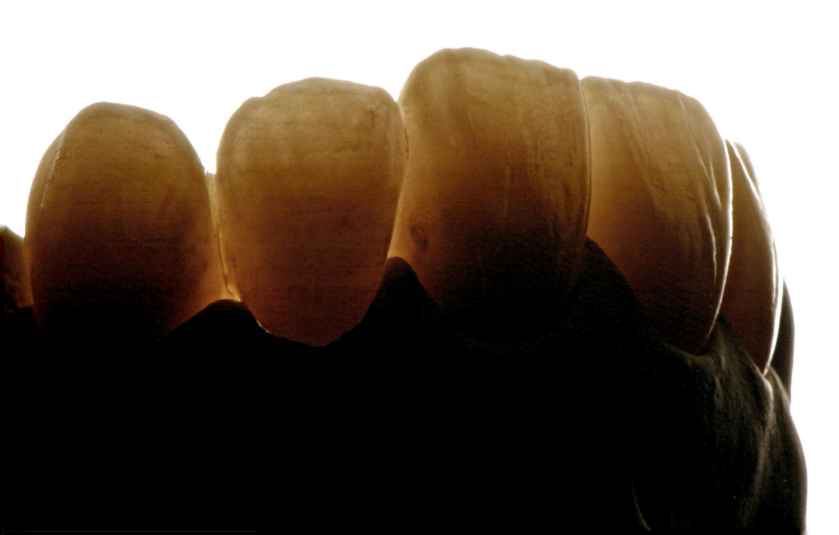

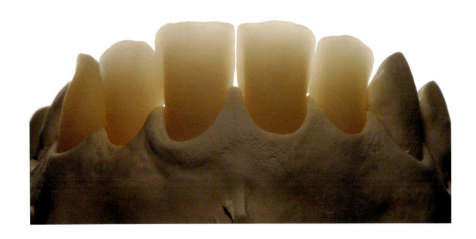

#7,8 IPS e.max Crown & #9-11 Three Unit Bridge

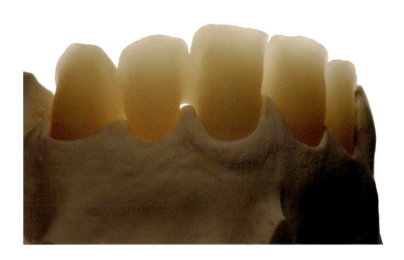

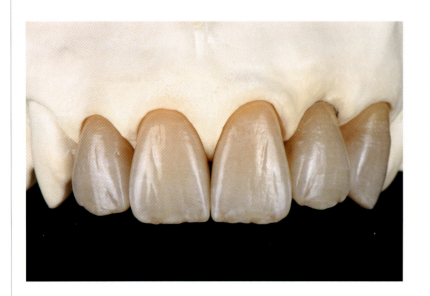
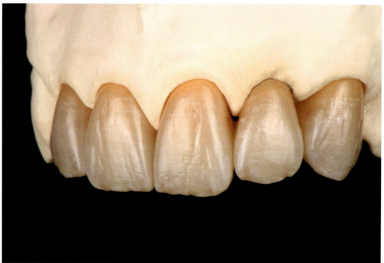

Exact Reproduction of Natural Dentition

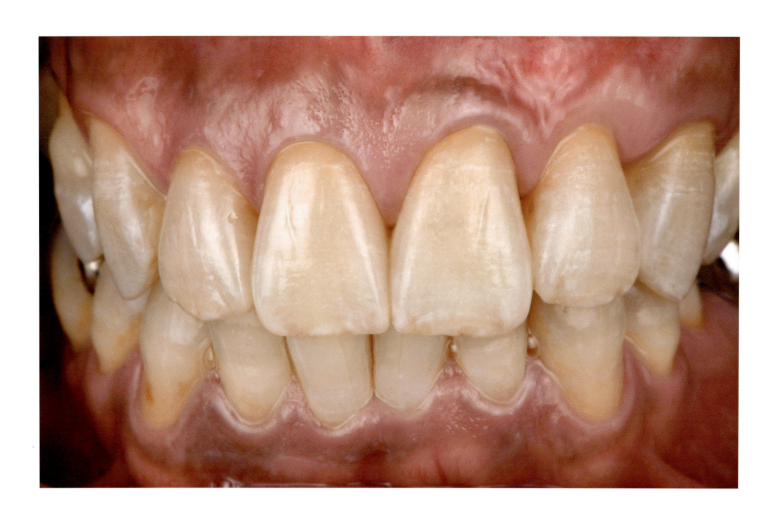

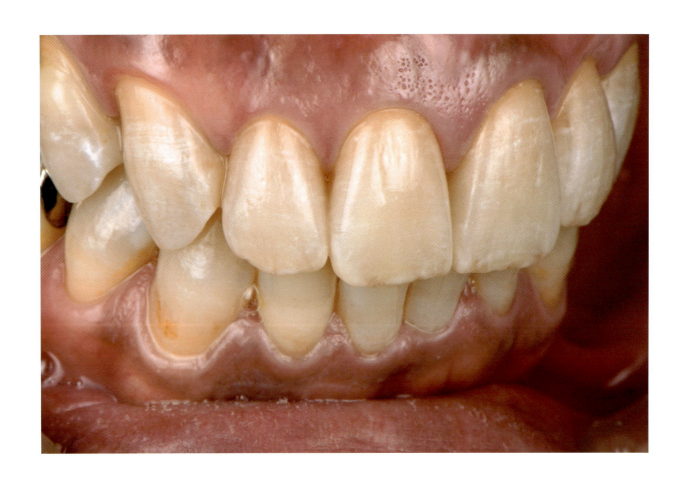

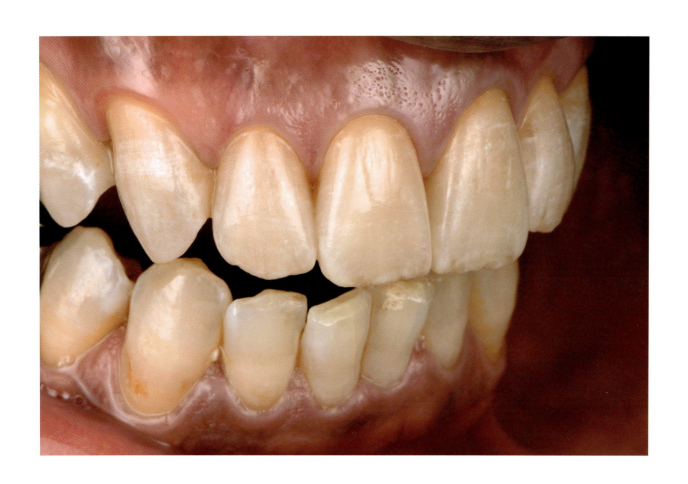

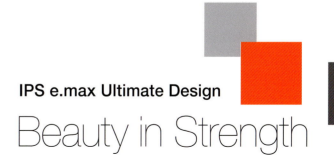

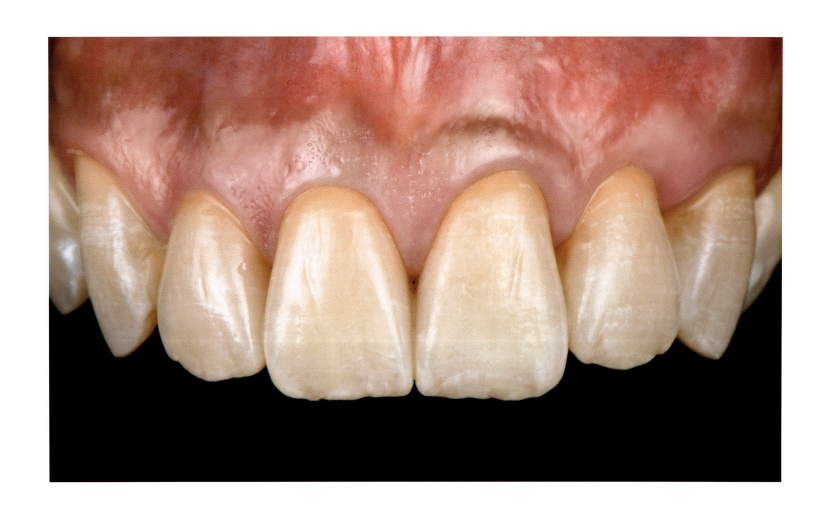

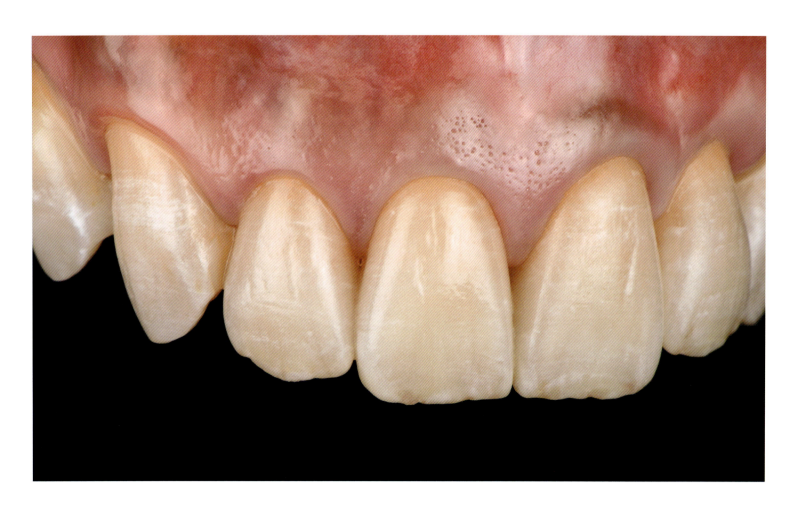

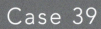

Case 39

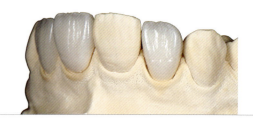

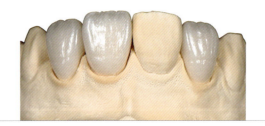

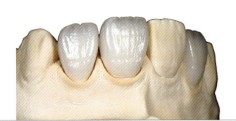

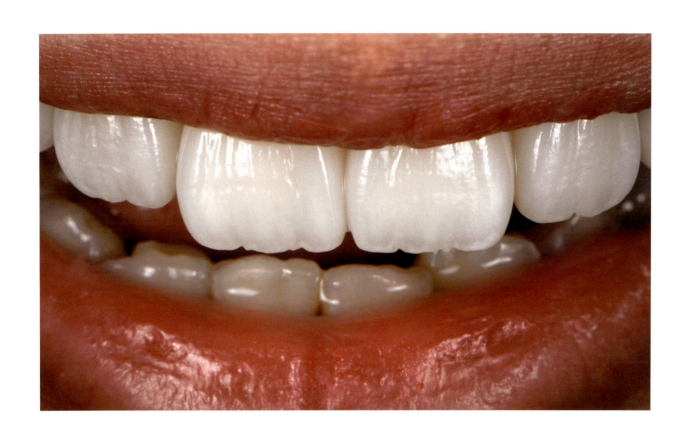

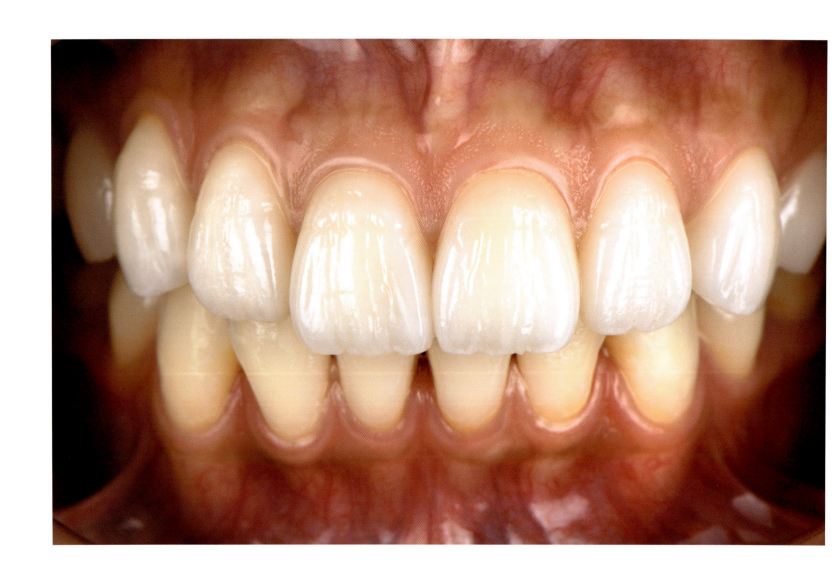

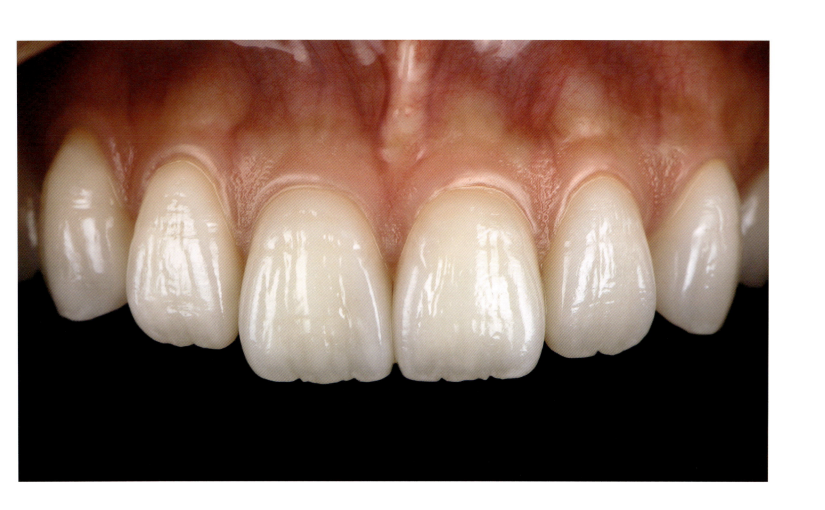

#6,7,9-11 IPS e.max Laminate Veneer & #5,8,12 IPS e.max Crown

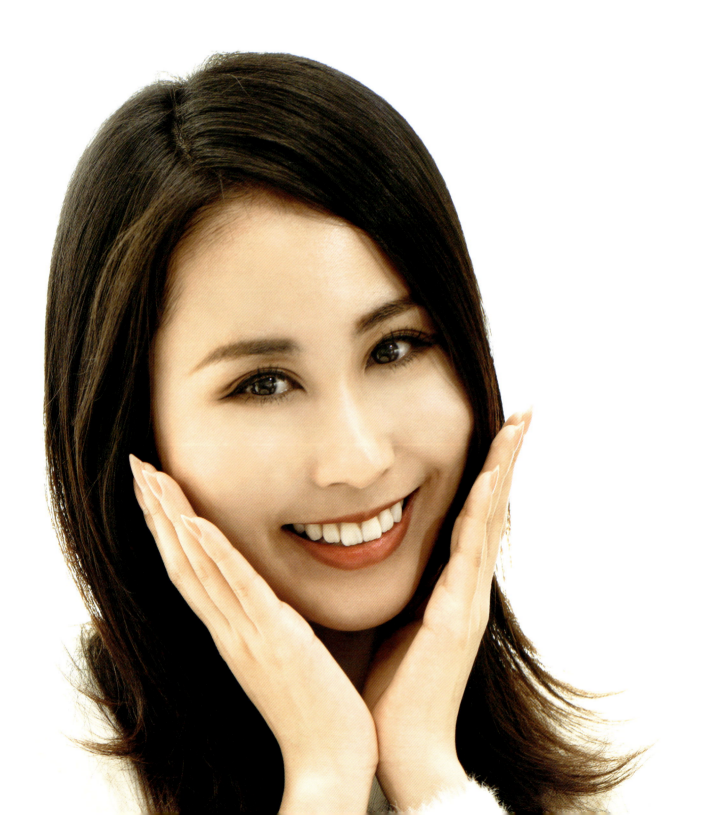

Smile Design

- It always makes us inspire -

Case 40

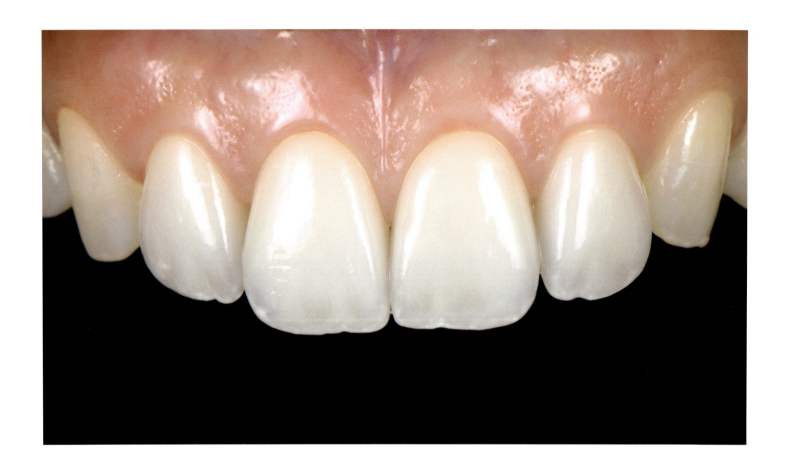

#7-10 IPS e.max Crown

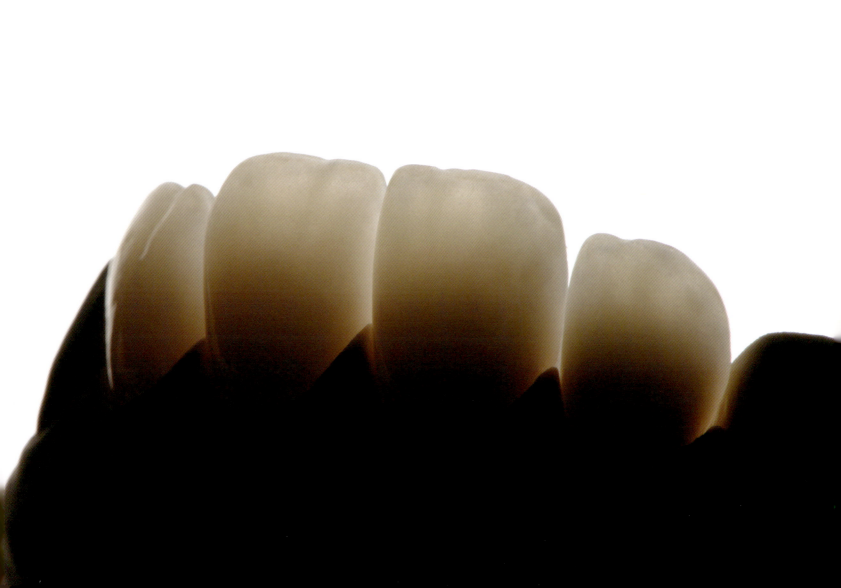

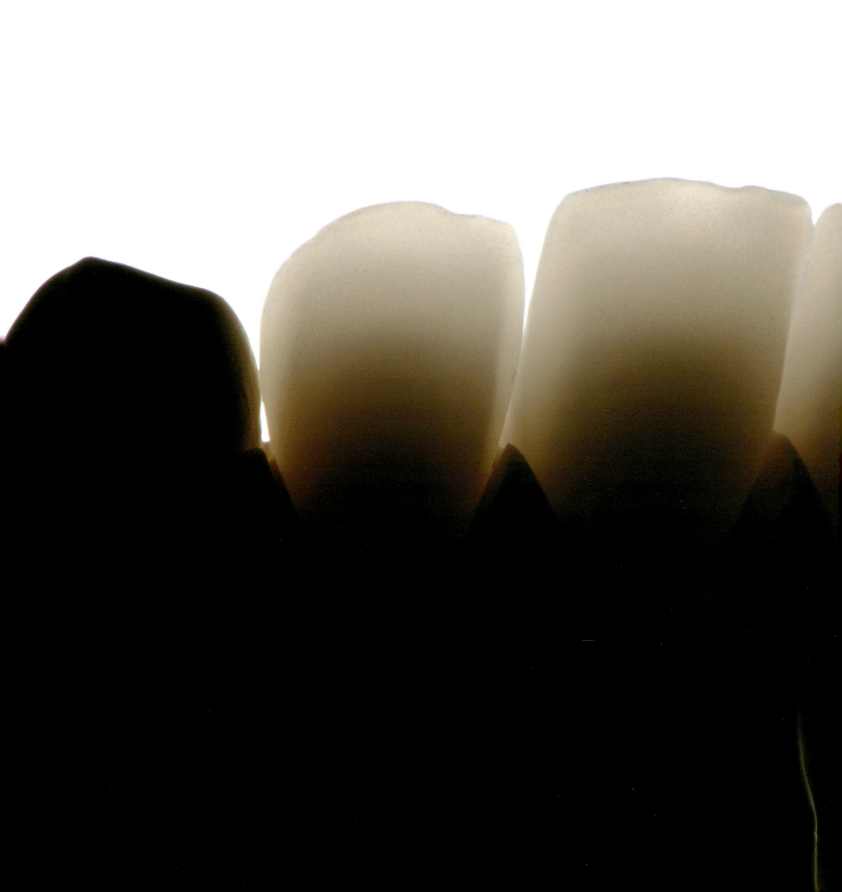

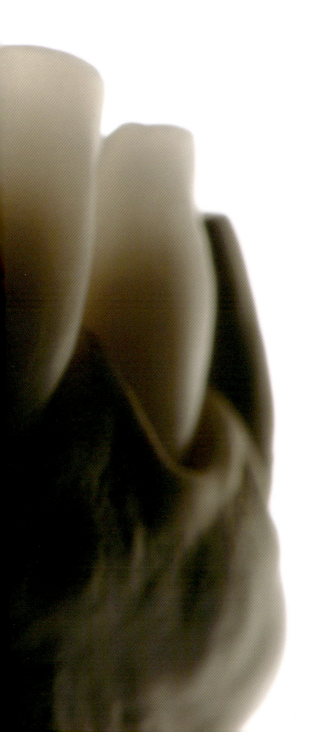

Beauty in Strength
IPS e.max Facial Cutback Design

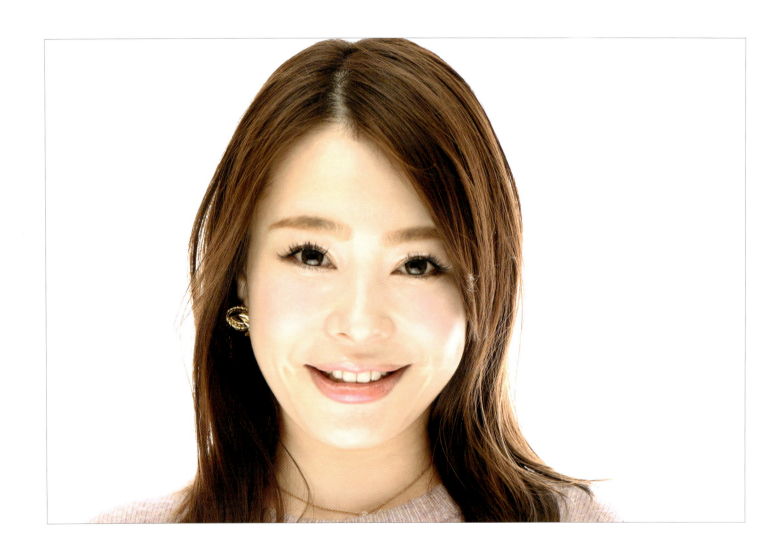

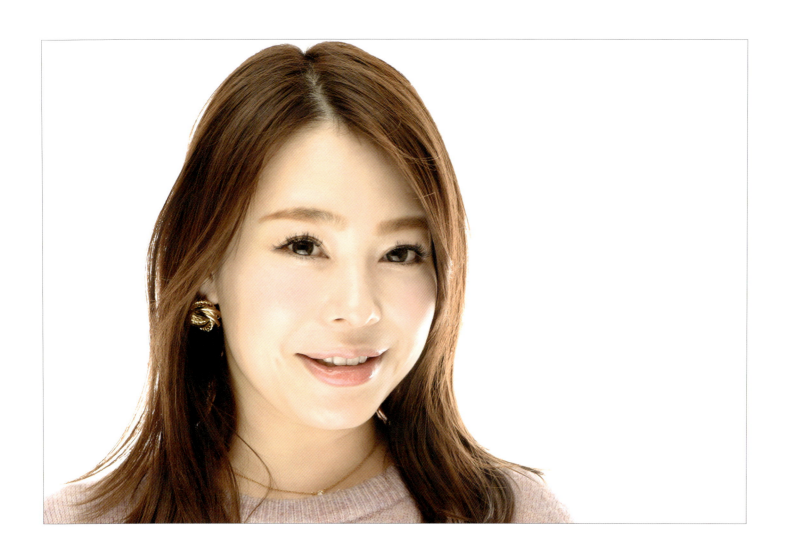

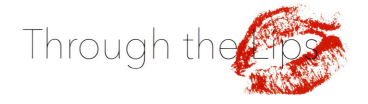

Through the Lips

Always follow your intuition

- Because there is a smile that can only be created by you -

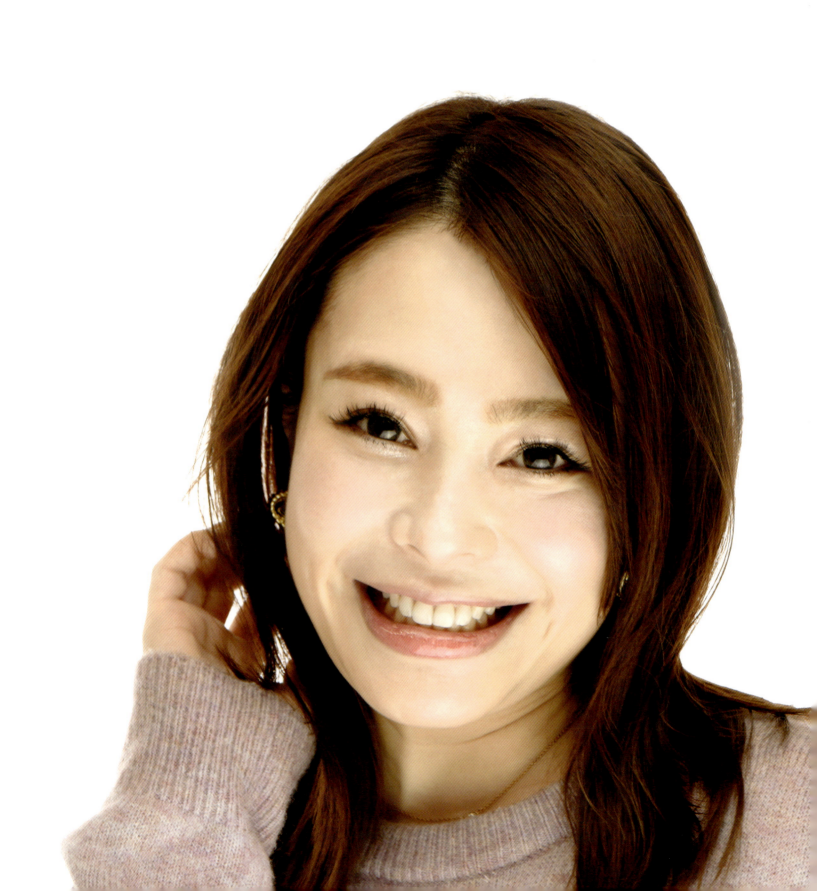

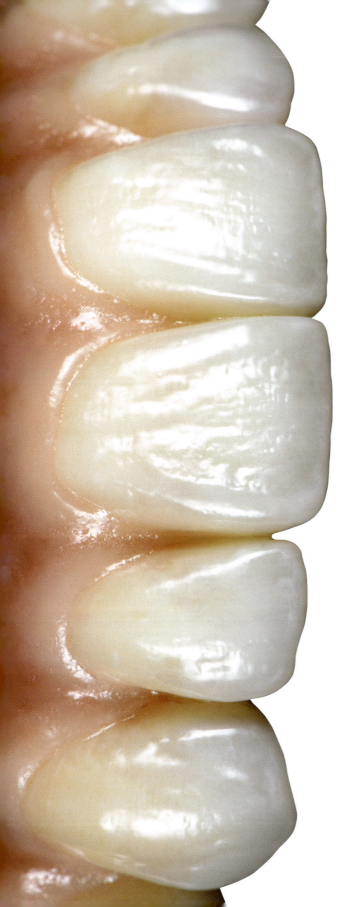

- Extra Case -

Full Mouse Reconstruction

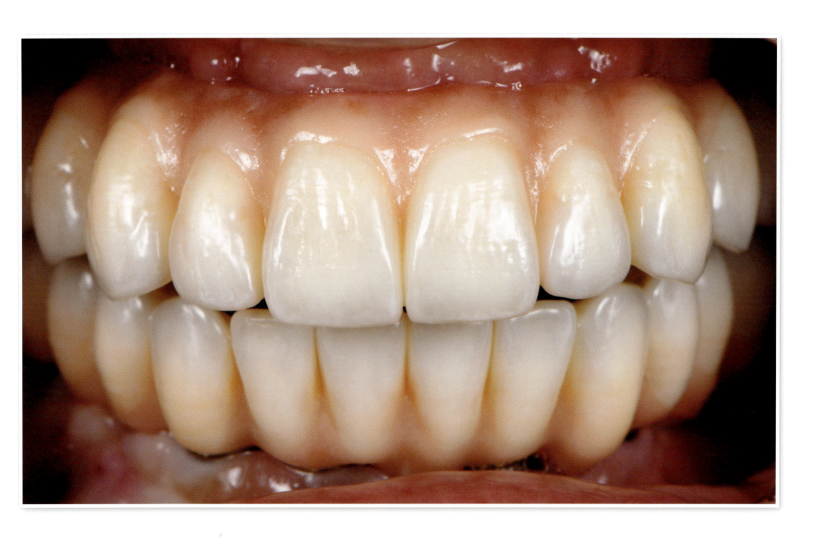

Always follow your intuition

- Because there is a smile that can only be created by you -

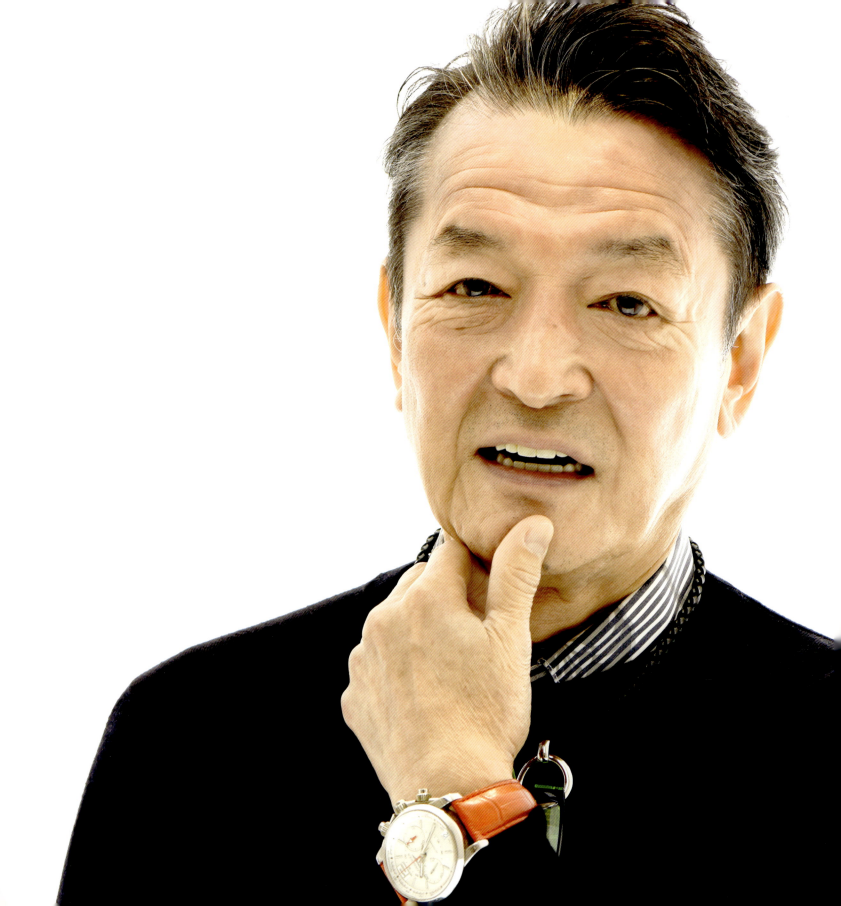

Ceramic Works I

- Breathing vivid life into new creations -

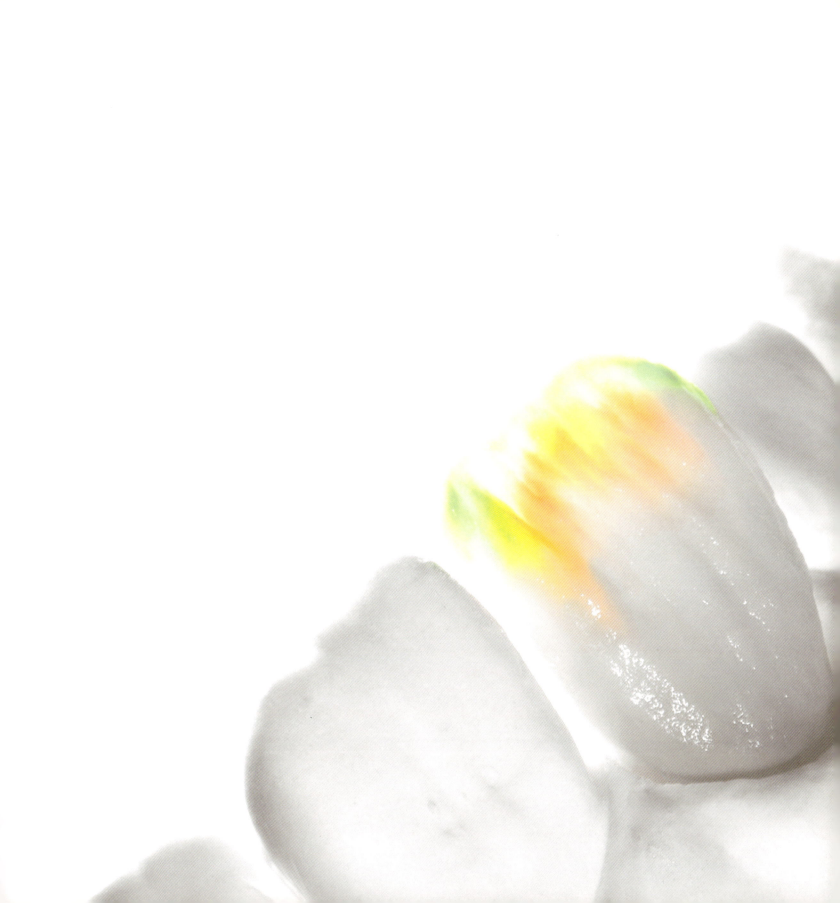

IPS e.max
Press & Layering
Technology

It has been enchanting you.

I. Target Shade

II. Material Selection

III. Ingot / Shade Selection

IV. Framework Design

IPS e.max Ceram

- Build up recipes -

Case 1

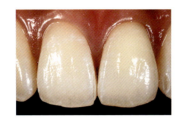

I. Target Shade — A2
II. Material Selection — IPS e.max Press
III. Ingot / Shade Selection — LT A1
IV. Framework Design — Anatomical Cutback Design

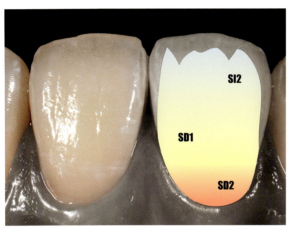

Foundation Stain

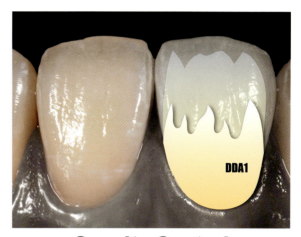

Opacity Control

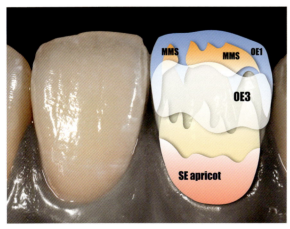

Internal Multi Layer

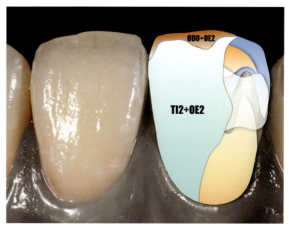

Enamel Skin Layer

Case 2

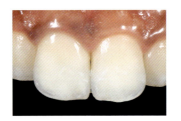

I. Target Shade — A2
II. Material Selection — IPS e.max Press
III. Ingot / Shade Selection — Impulse Opal1
IV. Framework Design — Facial Cutback Design

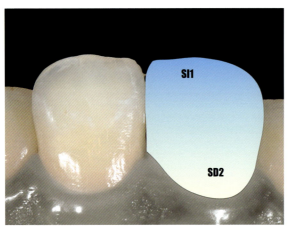

Foundation Stain

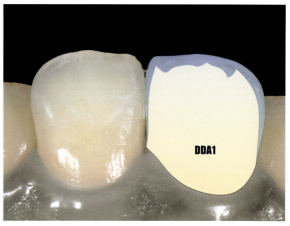

Opacity Control

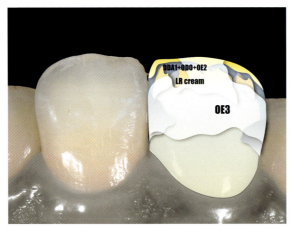

Internal Multi Layer

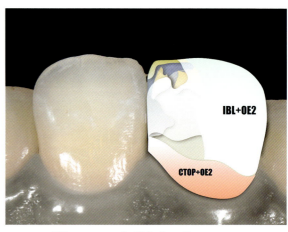

Enamel Skin Layer

Case 3

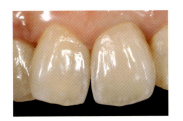

I. Target Shade — A3.5
II. Material Selection — IPS e.max Press
III. Ingot / Shade Selection — LT A3
IV. Framework Design — Anatomical Cutback Design

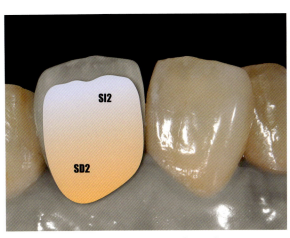

Foundation Stain

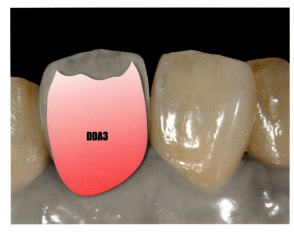

Opacity Control

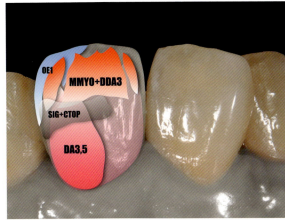

Internal Multi Layer

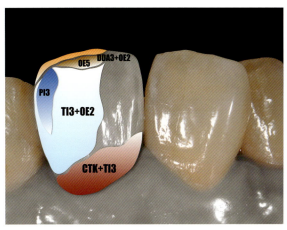

Enamel Skin Layer

Case 4

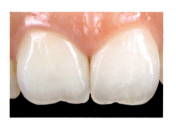

I. Target Shade	A2
II. Material Selection	IPS e.max Press
III. Ingot / Shade Selection	MO 1
IV. Framework Design	Full Coverage Design

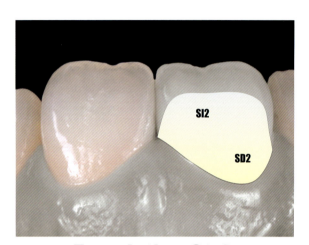

Foundation Stain

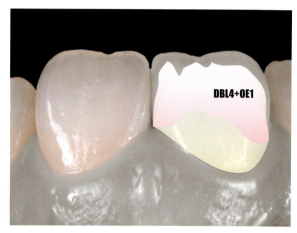

Opacity Control

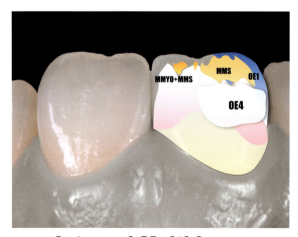

Internal Multi Layer

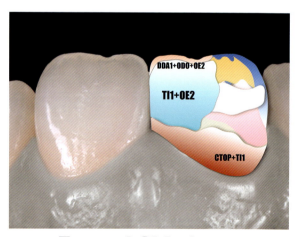

Enamel Skin Layer

Case 5

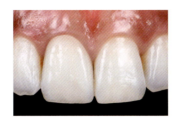

I. Target Shade — A2
II. Material Selection — IPS e.max Press
III. Ingot / Shade Selection — MO 0
IV. Framework Design — Full Coverage Design

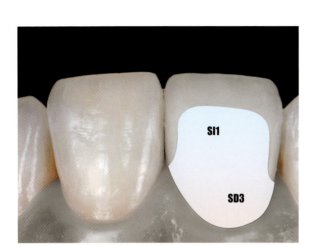

Foundation Stain

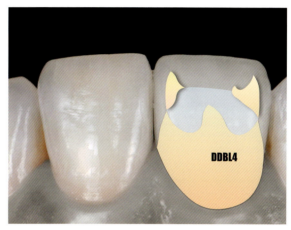

Opacity Control

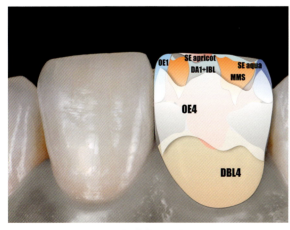

Internal Multi Layer

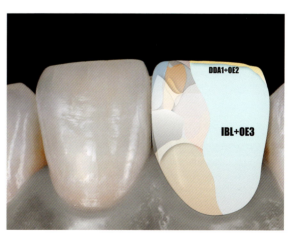

Enamel Skin Layer

Case 6

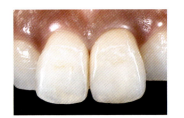

I. Target Shade — A3
II. Material Selection — IPS e.max Press
III. Ingot / Shade Selection — LT A1
IV. Framework Design — Anatomical Cutback Design

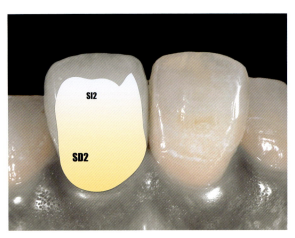

Foundation Stain

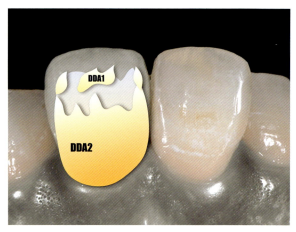

Opacity Control

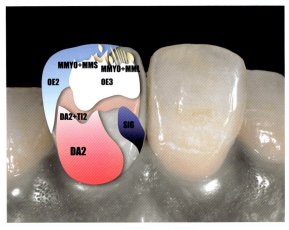

Internal Multi Layer

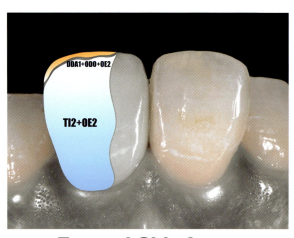

Enamel Skin Layer

Case 7

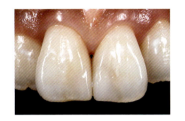

I. Target Shade — A3
II. Material Selection — IPS e.max Press
III. Ingot / Shade Selection — LT A1
IV. Framework Design — Anatomical Cutback Design

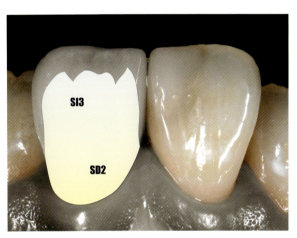
Foundation Stain

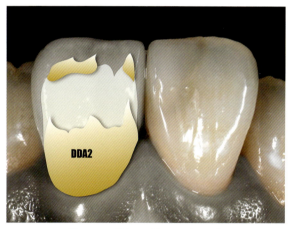
Opacity Control

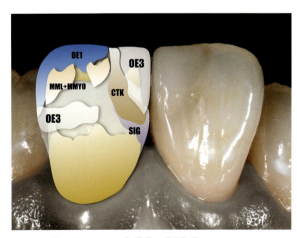
Internal Multi Layer

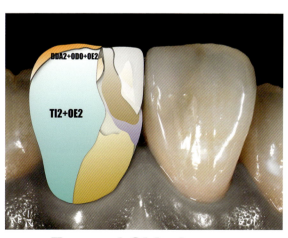
Enamel Skin Layer

Case 8

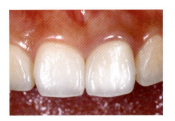

I. Target Shade — A2
II. Material Selection — IPS e.max Press
III. Ingot / Shade Selection — LT BL4
IV. Framework Design — Full Coverage Design

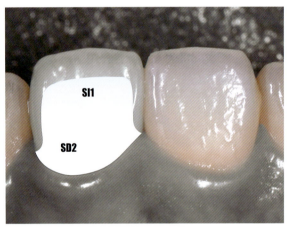

Foundation Stain

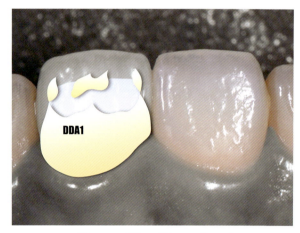

Opacity Control

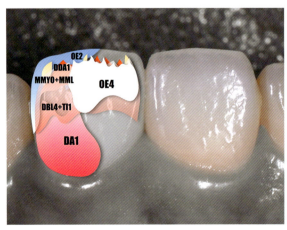

Internal Multi Layer

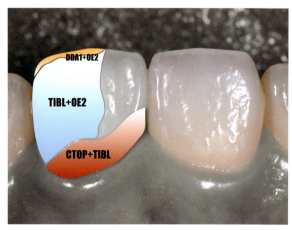

Enamel Skin Layer

Case 9

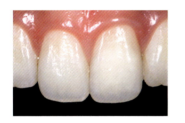

I. Target Shade — A2
II. Material Selection — IPS e.max Press
III. Ingot / Shade Selection — LT BL4
IV. Framework Design — Full Coverage Design

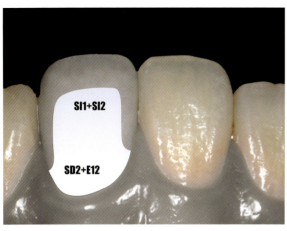

Foundation Stain

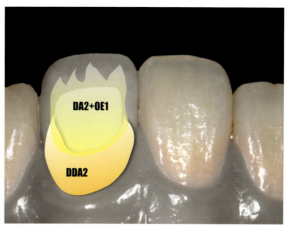

Opacity Control

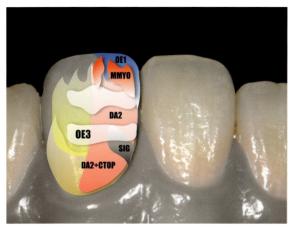

Internal Multi Layer

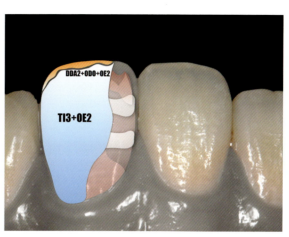

Enamel Skin Layer

Case 10

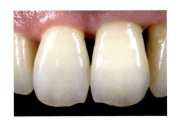

I. Target Shade — A3
II. Material Selection — IPS e.max Press
III. Ingot / Shade Selection — MT BL4
IV. Framework Design — Anatomical Cutback Design

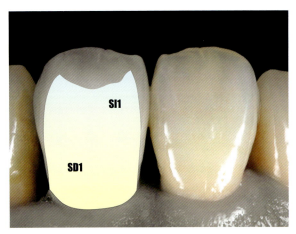

Foundation Stain

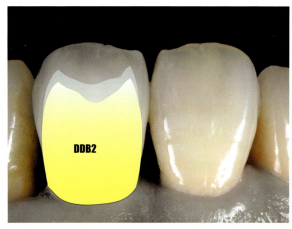

Opacity Control

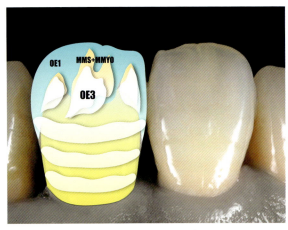

Internal Multi Layer

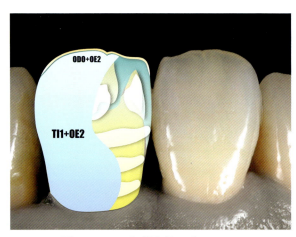

Enamel Skin Layer

Case 11

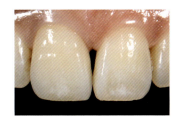

I. Target Shade — A3
II. Material Selection — IPS e.max Press
III. Ingot / Shade Selection — LT A1
IV. Framework Design — Facial Cutback Design

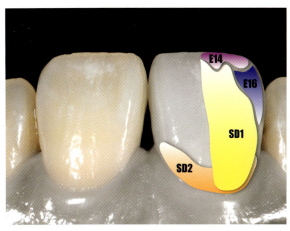

Foundation Stain

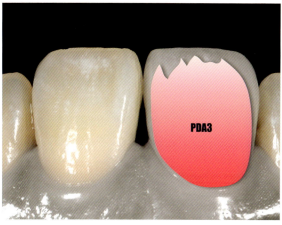

Opacity Control

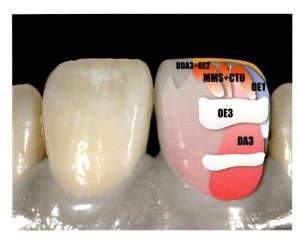

Internal Multi Layer

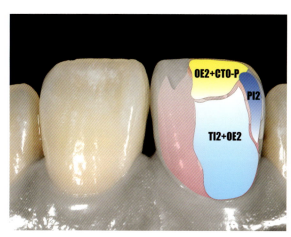

Enamel Skin Layer

Case 12

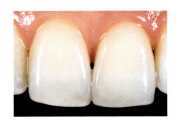

I. Target Shade — A2
II. Material Selection — IPS e.max Press
III. Ingot / Shade Selection — LT A1
IV. Framework Design — Anatomical Cutback Design

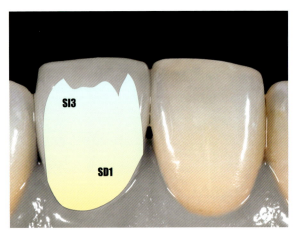

Foundation Stain

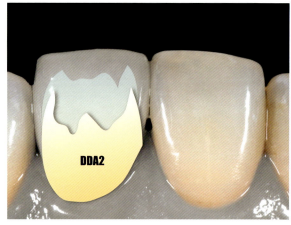

Opacity Control

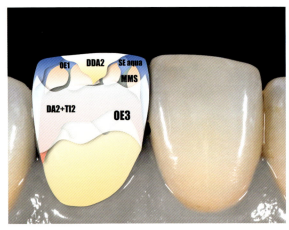

Internal Multi Layer

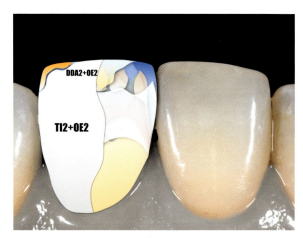

Enamel Skin Layer

Case 13

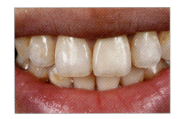

I. Target Shade — A2
II. Material Selection — IPS e.max Press
III. Ingot / Shade Selection — LT BL4
IV. Framework Design — Full Coverage Design

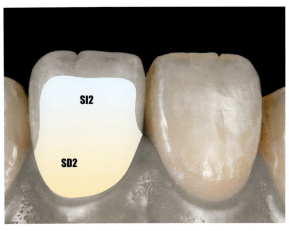

Foundation Stain

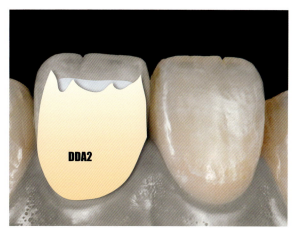

Opacity Control

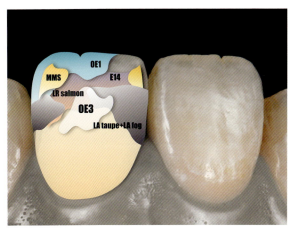

Internal Multi Layer

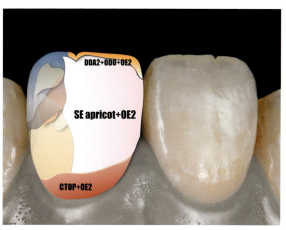

Enamel Skin Layer

Case 14

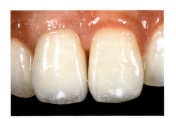

I. Target Shade — A3
II. Material Selection — IPS e.max ZirCAD
III. Ingot / Shade Selection — MO 0
IV. Framework Design — Full Coverage Design

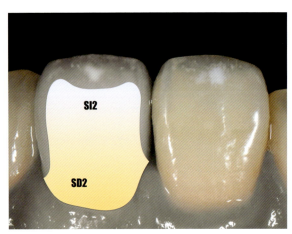

Foundation Stain

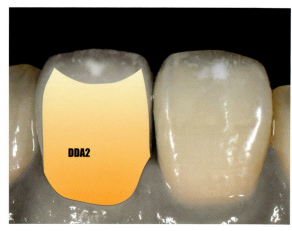

Opacity Control

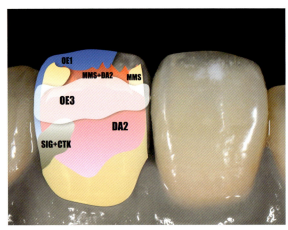

Internal Multi Layer

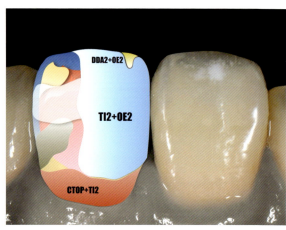

Enamel Skin Layer

Case 15

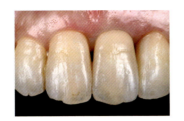

I. Target Shade — A3
II. Material Selection — IPS e.max Press
III. Ingot / Shade Selection — LT A1
IV. Framework Design — Anatomical Cutback Design

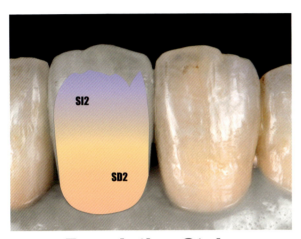

Foundation Stain

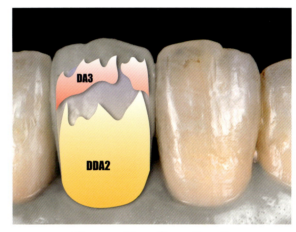

Opacity Control

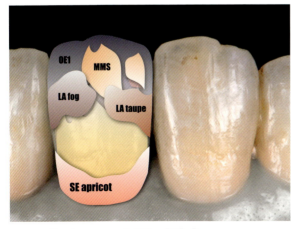

Internal Multi Layer

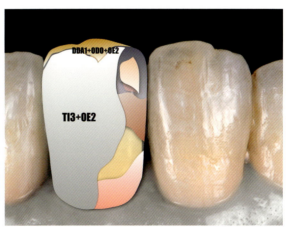

Enamel Skin Layer

Case 16

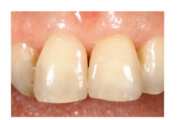

I. Target Shade — A3
II. Material Selection — IPS e.max Press
III. Ingot / Shade Selection — LT A1
IV. Framework Design — Facial Cutback Design

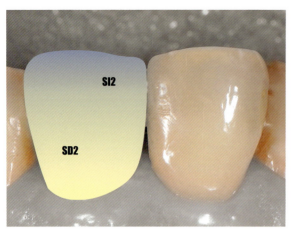

Foundation Stain

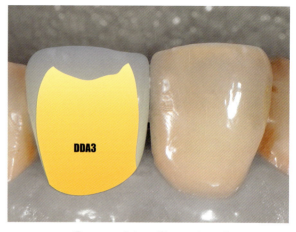

Opacity Control

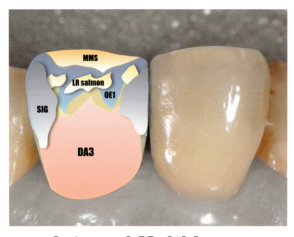

Internal Multi Layer

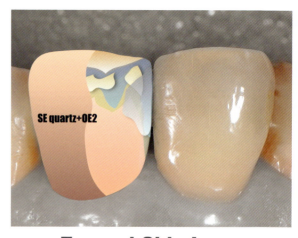

Enamel Skin Layer

Case 17

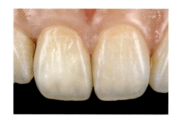

I. Target Shade — A2
II. Material Selection — IPS e.max Press
III. Ingot / Shade Selection — LT BL4
IV. Framework Design — Anatomical Cutback Design

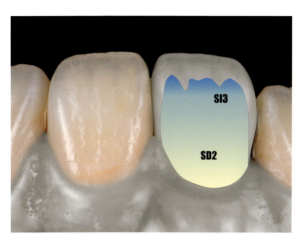

Foundation Stain

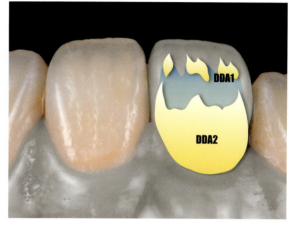

Opacity Control

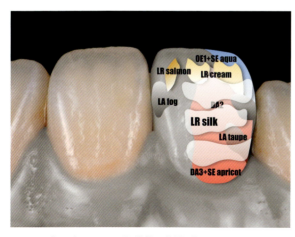

Internal Multi Layer

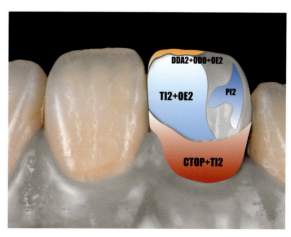

Enamel Skin Layer

Case 18

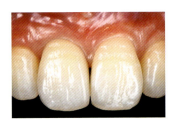

I. Target Shade — B3
II. Material Selection — IPS e.max ZirCAD
III. Ingot / Shade Selection — MT Multi B1
IV. Framework Design — Facial Cutback Design

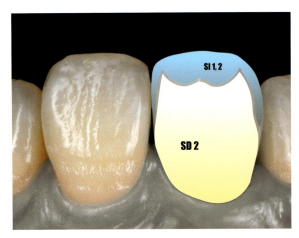

Foundation Stain

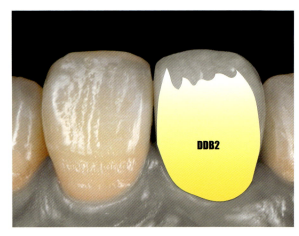

Opacity Control

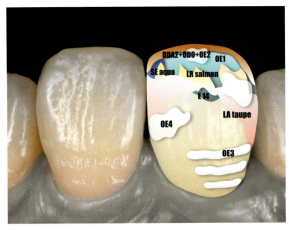

Internal Multi Layer

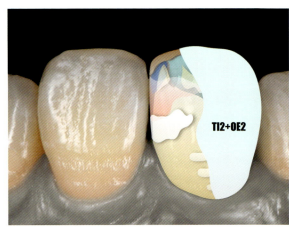

Enamel Skin Layer

Case 27

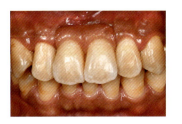

I. Target Shade	A3.5
II. Material Selection	Zirconia
III. Ingot / Shade Selection	Zenostar Sun
IV. Framework Design	Anatomical Cutback Design

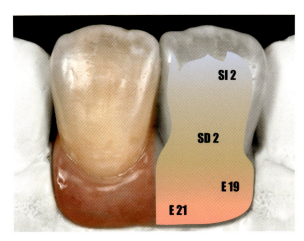

Foundation Stain

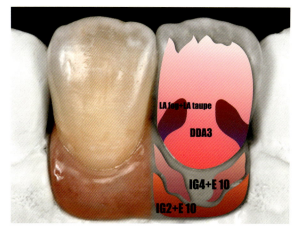

Opacity Control

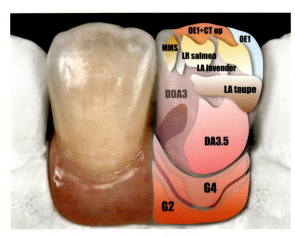

Internal Multi Layer

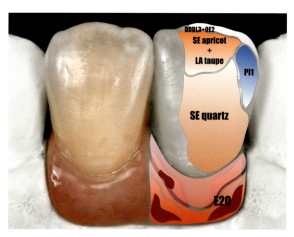

Enamel Skin Layer

Case 29

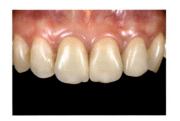

I. Target Shade — A3.5
II. Material Selection — Zirconia
III. Ingot / Shade Selection — Zenostar Sun
IV. Framework Design — Anatomical Cutback Design

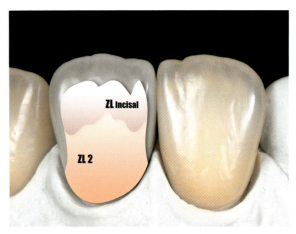

Foundation Stain

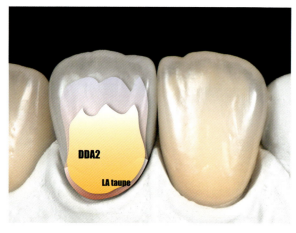

Opacity Control

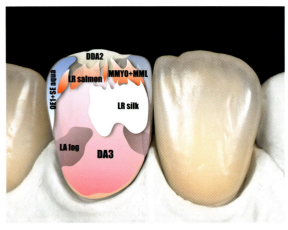

Internal Multi Layer

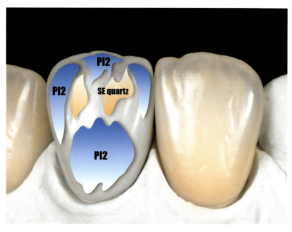

Enamel Skin Layer

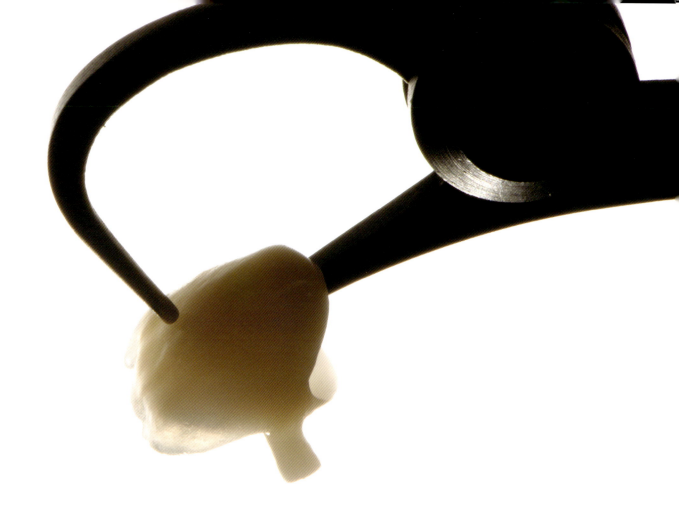

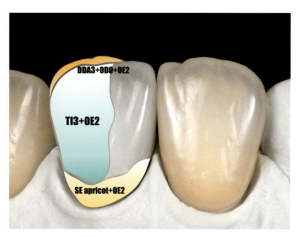

Enamel Skin Layer

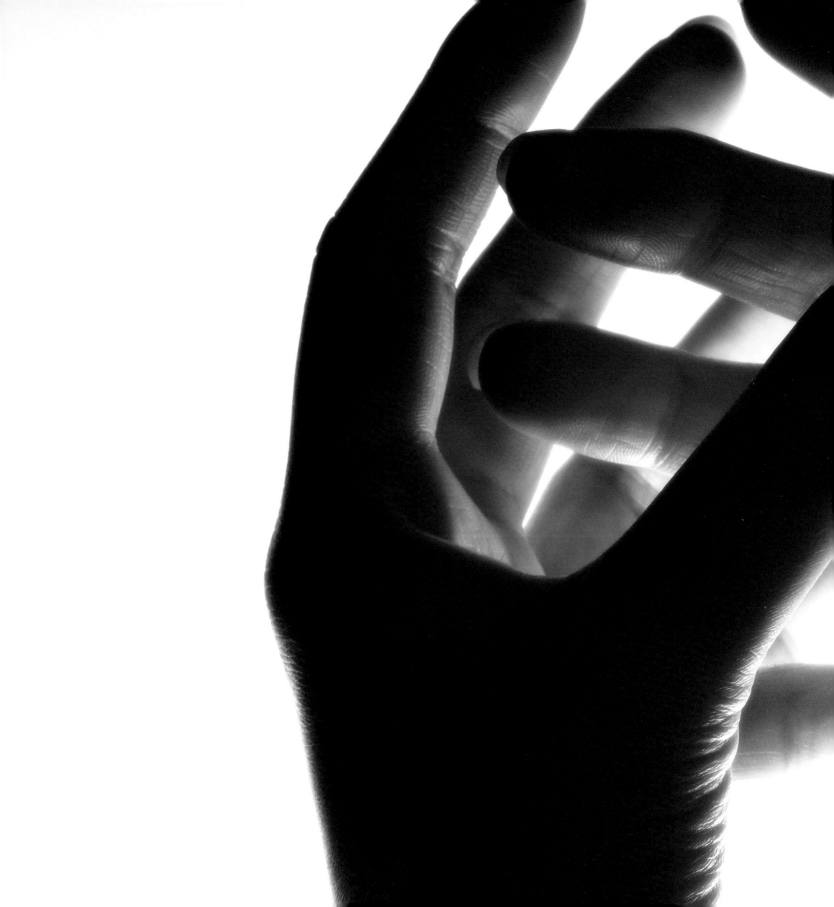

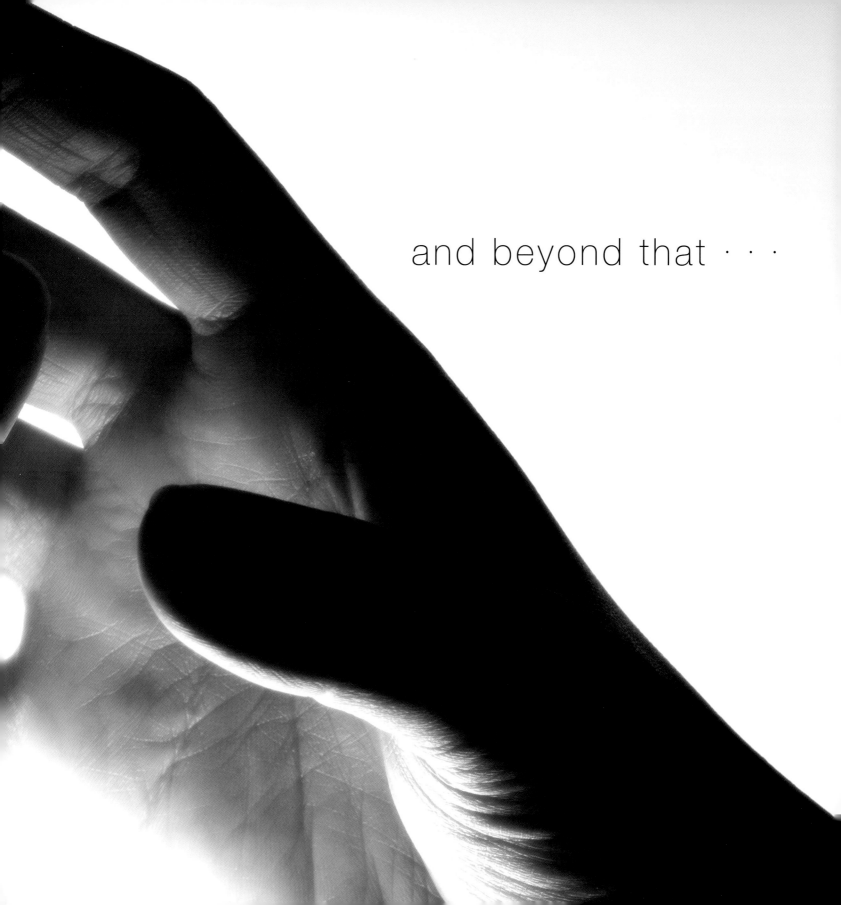
and beyond that · · ·

- Behind the scenes -

Collaboration & Partnership

Case 1

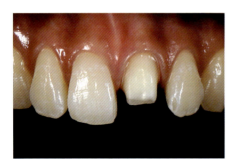

Restoration: #9
Material: IPS e.max Press
Application: IPS e.max Ceram
Technology: Layering Technique
Dentist: Dr.Tsutomu Kubota

Case 2

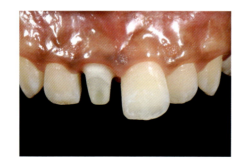

Restoration: #8
Material: IPS e.max Press
Application: IPS e.max Ceram
Technology: Layering Technique
Dentist: Dr.Yusuke Yamaguchi

Case 3

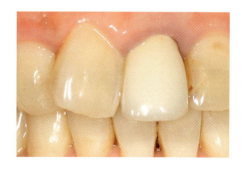

Restoration: #9
Material: IPS e.max Press
Application: IPS e.max Ceram
Technology: Layering Technique
Dentist: Dr.Hiroyuki Takino

Case 4

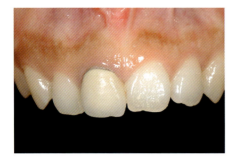

Restoration: #8
Material: IPS e.max Press
Application: IPS e.max Ceram
Technology: Layering Technique
Dentist: Dr.Hirofumi Takai

Case 5

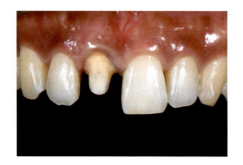

Restoration: #8
Material: IPS e.max Press
Application: IPS e.max Ceram
Technology: Layering Technique
Dentist: Dr.Hiroyuki Takino

Case 6

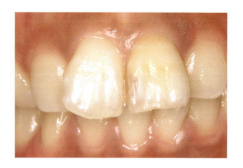

Restoration: #9
Material: IPS e.max Press
Application: IPS e.max Ceram
Technology: Layering Technique
Dentist: Dr.Yusuke Yamaguchi

Case 7

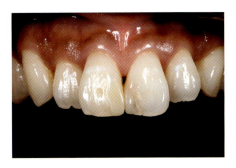

Restoration: #8
Material: IPS e.max Press
Application: IPS e.max Ceram
Technology: Layering Technique
Dentist: Dr.Tsutomu Kubota

Case 8

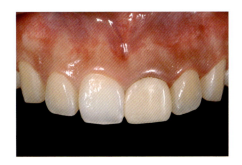

Restoration: #9
Material: IPS e.max Press
Application: IPS e.max Ceram
Technology: Layering Technique
Dentist: Dr.Hiroyuki Takino

Case 9

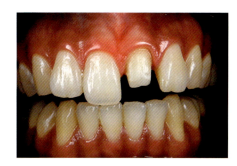

Restoration: #9
Material: IPS e.max Press
Application: IPS e.max Ceram
Technology: Layering Technique
Dentist: Dr.Tsutomu Kubota

Case 10

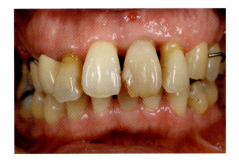

Restoration: #7,9
Material: IPS e.max Press
Application: IPS e.max Ceram
Technology: Layering Technique
Dentist: Dr.Tsutomu Kubota

Case 11

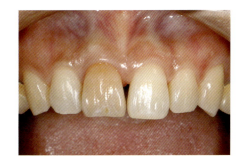

Restoration: #8
Material: IPS e.max Press
Application: IPS e.max Ceram
Technology: Layering Technique
Dentist: Dr.Tsutomu Kubota

Case 12

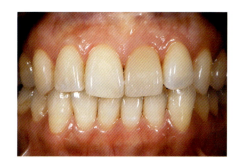

Restoration: #9
Material: IPS e.max Press
Application: IPS e.max Ceram
Technology: Layering Technique
Dentist: Dr.Tsutomu Kubota

Case 13

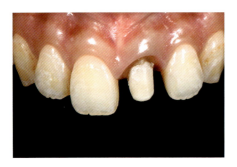

Restoration: #9
Material: IPS e.max Press
Application: IPS e.max Ceram
Technology: Layering Technique
Dentist: Dr.Yuya Iwasaki

Case 14

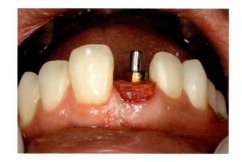

Restoration: #8
Material: IPS e.max ZirCAD
Application: IPS e.max Ceram
Technology: Layering Technique
Dentist: Dr.Tatsunori Nagao

Case 15

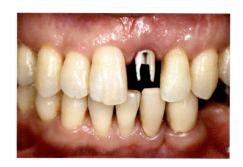

Restoration: #9
Material: IPS e.max Press
Application: IPS e.max Ceram
Technology: Layering Technique
Dentist: Dr.Hiroyuki Takino

Case 16

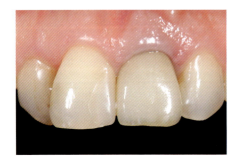

Restoration: #9
Material: IPS e.max Press
Application: IPS e.max Ceram
Technology: Layering Technique
Dentist: Dr.Tetsunari Hongo

Case 17

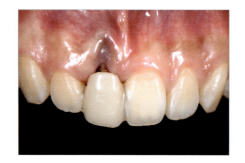

Restoration: #8
Material: IPS e.max Press
Application: IPS e.max Ceram
Technology: Layering Technique
Dentist: Dr.Hiroyuki Takino

Case 18

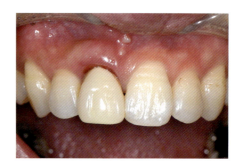

Restoration: #8
Material: IPS e.max ZirCAD
Application: IPS e.max Ceram
Technology: Layering Technique
Dentist: Dr.Hiroyuki Takino

Case 19

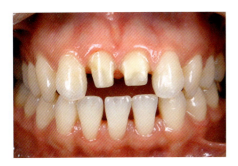

Restoration: #8,9
Material: IPS e.max Press
Application: IPS e.max Ceram
Technology: Layering Technique
Dentist: Dr.Hidenori Sasaki

Case 20

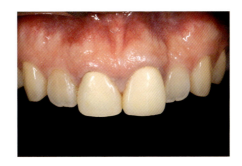

Restoration: #8,9
Material: IPS e.max Press
Application: IPS e.max Ceram
Technology: Layering Technique
Dentist: Dr.Yusuke Yamaguchi

Case 21

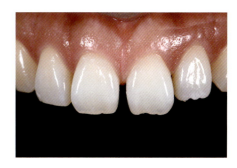

Restoration: #8,9
Material: IPS e.max Press
Application: IPS Ivocolor
Technology: Staining Technique
Dentist: Dr.Hiroyuki Takino

Case 22

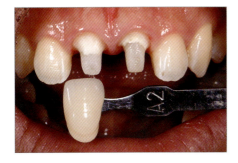

Restoration: #8,9
Material: IPS e.max Press
Application: IPS e.max Ceram
Technology: Layering Technique
Dentist: Dr.Hiroyuki Takino

Case 23

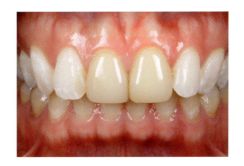

Restoration: #8,9
Material: IPS e.max Press
Application: IPS Ivocolor
Technology: Staining Technique
Dentist: Dr.Naohisa Okamoto

Case 24

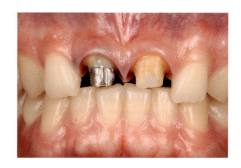

Restoration: #8,9
Material: IPS e.max Press
Application: IPS Ivocolor
Technology: Staining Technique
Dentist: Dr.Tsutomu Kubota

Case 25

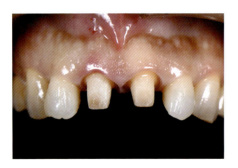

Restoration: #8,9
Material: IPS e.max Press
Application: IPS e.max Ceram
Technology: Layering Technique
Dentist: Dr.Yusuke Yamaguchi

Case 26

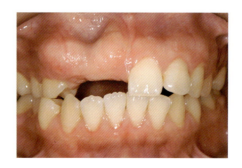

Restoration: #8,9
Material: IPS e.max Press
Application: IPS Ivocolor
Technology: Staining Technique
Dentist: Dr.Hiroyuki Takino

Case 27

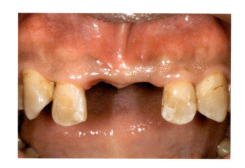

Restoration: #8,9
Material: Zenostar Sun
Application: IPS e.max Ceram
Technology: Layering Technique
Dentist: Dr.Hiroyuki Takino

Case 28

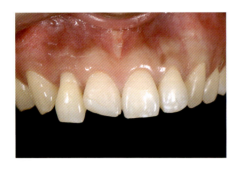

Restoration: #7,8
Material: IPS e.max Press
Application: IPS e.max Ceram
Technology: Layering Technique
Dentist: Dr.Hiroyuki Takino

Case 29

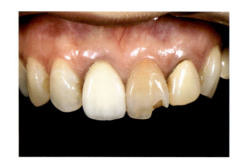

Restoration: #8-10
Material: Zenostar Sun
Application: IPS e.max Ceram
Technology: Layering Technique
Dentist: Dr.Tsutomu Kubota

Case 30

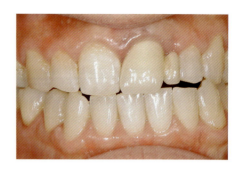

Restoration: #8-10
Material: IPS e.max Press
Application: IPS e.max Ceram
Technology: Layering & Staining
Dentist: Dr.Toru Yamaba

Case 31

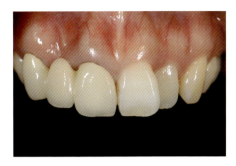

Restoration: #6-8
Material: IPS e.max Press
Application: IPS e.max Ceram
Technology: Layering Technique
Dentist: Dr.Hiroyuki Takino

Case 32

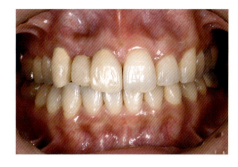

Restoration: #6-8
Material: IPS e.max Press
Application: IPS e.max Ceram
Technology: Layering Technique
Dentist: Dr.Hiroyuki Takino

Case 33

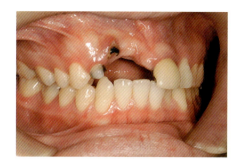

Restoration: #6-8
Material: Zenostar Pure
Application: IPS e.max Ceram
Technology: Layering Technique
Dentist: Dr.Hiroyuki Takino

Case 34

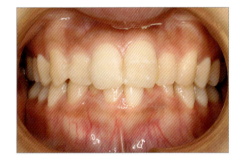

Restoration: #7-10
Material: IPS e.max Press
Application: IPS Ivocolor, e.max Ceram
Technology: Layering & Staining
Dentist: Dr.Tatsunori Nagao

Case 35

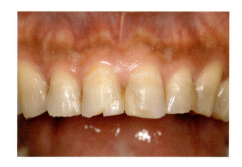

Restoration: #7-10
Material: IPS e.max Press
Application: IPS e.max Ceram
Technology: Layering Technique
Dentist: Dr.Tsutomu Kubota

Case 36

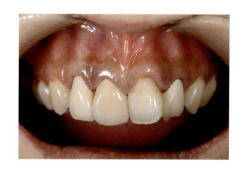

Restoration: #7-10
Material: IPS e.max Press
Application: IPS e.max Ceram
Technology: Layering Technique
Dentist: Dr.Hiroyuki Takino

Case 37

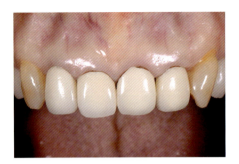

Restoration: #7-10
Material: IPS e.max Press
Application: IPS e.max Ceram
Technology: Layering Technique
Dentist: Dr.Yusuke Yamaguchi

Case 38

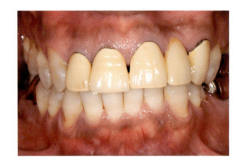

Restoration: #7-11
Material: IPS e.max Press
Application: IPS e.max Ceram
Technology: Layering Technique
Dentist: Dr.Yusuke Yamaguchi

Case 39

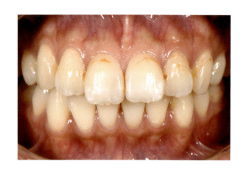

Restoration: #5-12
Material: IPS e.max Press
Application: IPS e.max Ceram
Technology: Layering Technique
Dentist: Dr.Tsutomu Kubota

Case 40

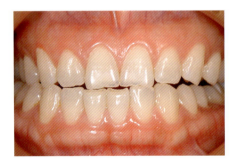

Restoration: #7-10
Material: IPS e.max Press
Application: IPS e.max Ceram
Technology: Layering Technique
Dentist: Dr.Makoto Ono

The Best For You

IPS e.max solutions

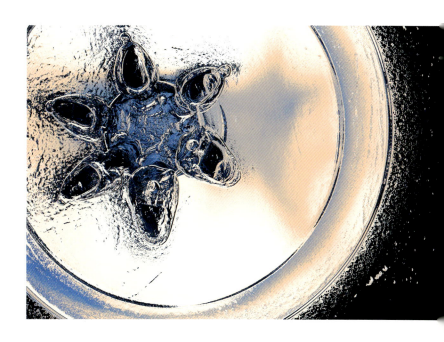

Epilogue

笑顔をつくる仕事

そこには情熱をそそぐ価値がある

あなたにしかつくれない笑顔があるから

だから１つでも多くの笑顔を届けたい

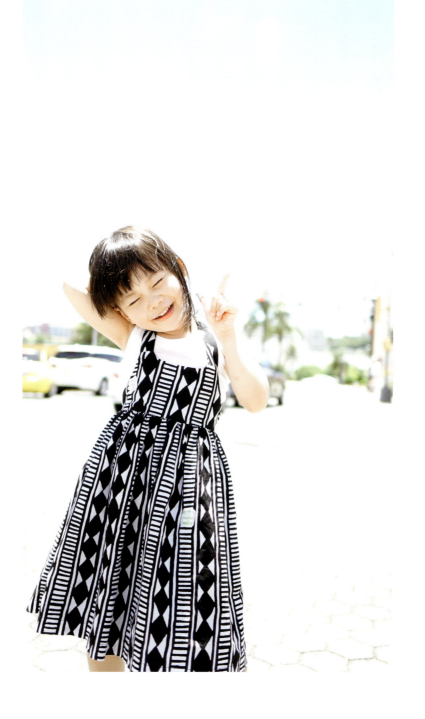

【著者略歴】

都築 優治
つづき ゆうじ

2001年　新大阪歯科技工士専門学校 専攻科卒業
2005年　茂野歯科医院 勤務
2007年　伊藤歯科医院 勤務
2009年　Ray Dental Labor 開業
　　　　Ivoclar Vivadent 公認インストラクター
　　　　Clinical Enhancement Course 主宰

envisage think what can be

ISBN978-4-263-46148-8

2019年 6 月 25 日　第 1 版第 1 刷発行

著　者　都　築　優　治
発行者　白　石　泰　夫

発行所　医歯薬出版株式会社

〒113-8612　東京都文京区本駒込 1-7-10
TEL.（03）5395-7635（編集）・7630（販売）
FAX.（03）5395-7639（編集）・7633（販売）
　　　　http://www.ishiyaku.co.jp/
郵便振替番号　00190-5-13816

乱丁・落丁の際はお取り替えいたします　　印刷・第一印刷所／製本・第一印刷所
© Ishiyaku Publishers, Inc., 2019. Printed in Japan

本書の複製権・翻訳権・翻案権・上映権・譲渡権・貸与権・公衆送信権（送信可能化権を含む）・口述権は，医歯薬出版㈱が保有します．
本書を無断で複製する行為（コピー，スキャン，デジタルデータ化など）は，「私的使用のための複製」などの著作権法上の限られた例外を除き禁じられています．また私的使用に該当する場合であっても，請負業者等の第三者に依頼し上記の行為を行うことは違法となります．

JCOPY ＜(社)出版者著作権管理機構 委託出版物＞
本書をコピーやスキャン等により複製される場合は，そのつど事前に(社)出版者著作権管理機構（電話 03-5244-5088，FAX 03-5244-5089，e-mail: info@jcopy.or.jp）の許諾を得てください．